VAGUS NERVE

A HEALING POWER GUIDE WITH DAILY PRACTICAL EXERCISES TO ACTIVATE YOUR VAGUS NERVE. REDUCE DEPRESSION, ANXIETY, TRAUMA, PTSD, RELIEVE CHRONIC ILLNESS, INFLAMMATION AND STRESS.

Dr. JASON ROSENBERG

VAGUS NERVE

Copyright 2020 by Dr. JASON ROSENBERG - All rights reserved.

This content is provided with the sole purpose of providing relevant information on a specific topic for which every reasonable effort has been made to ensure that it is both accurate and reasonable. Nevertheless, by purchasing this content, you consent to the fact that the author, as well as the publisher, are in no way experts on the topics contained herein, regardless of any claims as such that may be made within. As such, any suggestions or recommendations that are made within are done so purely for entertainment value. It is recommended that you always consult a professional prior to undertaking any of the advice or techniques discussed within.

This is a legally binding declaration that is considered both valid and fair by both the Committee of Publishers Association and the American Bar Association and should be considered as legally binding within the United States.

The reproduction, transmission, and duplication of any of the content found herein, including any specific or extended information, will be done as an illegal act regardless of the end form the information ultimately takes. This includes copied versions of the work, both physical, digital, and audio unless express consent of the Publisher is provided beforehand. Any additional rights reserved.

Furthermore, the information that can be found within the pages described forthwith shall be considered both accurate and truthful when it comes to the recounting of facts. As such, any use, correct or incorrect, of the provided information will render the Publisher free of responsibility as to the actions taken outside of their direct purview. Regardless, there are zero scenarios where the original author or the Publisher can be deemed liable in any fashion for any damages or hardships that may result from any of the information discussed herein.

Additionally, the information in the following pages is intended only for informational purposes and should thus be thought of as universal. As befitting its nature, it is presented without assurance regarding its prolonged validity or interim quality. Trademarks that are mentioned are done without written consent and can in no way be considered an endorsement from the trademark holder.

Dr. Jason Rosenberg

Table of Contents

- INTRODUCTION 1
- WHAT IS THE VAGUS NERVE? 5
- UNDERSTANDING POLYVAGAL THEORY: EMOTIONAL SHUTDOWN 13
- VAGUS NERVE ANATOMY AND FUNCTIONS 21
- 12 CRANIAL NERVE 33
- FUNCTIONS OF THE VAGUS NERVE 51
- ADVANTAGES AND TRUTH ABOUT VAGUS NERVE 59
- PTSD 75
- VAGUS NERVE – MENTAL HEALTH AND OTHER HEALTH ISSUES. 87
- THE NERVOUS SYSTEM 103
- CAUSES OF ANXIETY, DEPRESSION, AND INFLAMMATION 115
- WHAT HAPPENS IF THE VAGUS NERVE IS DAMAGED? 127
- ACTIVATING THE VAGUS NERVE 139
- ALTERNATIVE WAYS TO ACTIVATE VAGUS NERVE 147
- EXERCISES FOR THE VAGUS NERVE 155
- CONCLUSION 167

INTRODUCTION

Simply put, the vagus nerve is the supreme commander of your inner nerve center and regulates all your major organs. This is the longest ever cranial that starts behind the ears in the brain and interacts with all major bodies. This sends fibers, and actually directs the inner core of your nerve, to all your visceral organs, sending nerve impulses to every organ in your body. The term vagus means, basically, "hiking" because it stretches from the brain to the reproductive organs all over the body. The vagus nerve, except the surrender and thyroid glands, is important in connection with the mental body as it passes all major organs.

For each organ, it is in contact; this is an essential nerve. It helps prevent anxiety and depression in the brain. The reason for our response to each other is closely connected to the vaguely attached nervous system that adapts our ore to speak and coordinates eye contact and gestures. This nerve can also affect the correct release

VAGUS NERVE

of hormones in the body to maintain a healthy mind and body system.

The vagus nerve increases the acidity of the stomach and digestive juice production to promote digestion in the stomach. It can also help you absorb vitamin B12 when activated. If it does not work properly, you can then expect serious intestinal problems like Colitis, IBS, and Re-flux, only to name a few. Re-flux problems are caused by a vagus nerve problem because the esophagus is also regulated. It is the insufficient esophagus reflection that triggers conditions such as Gerd and Re-flux.

The vagus nerve also helps to prevent heart rate and blood pressure. In the liver and pancreas, the balance of blood glucose, avoiding diabetes, is regulated by this nerve. The vagus nerve helps to release bile when it travels through the gallbladder, which allows the body to absorb toxins and split fat. In the bladder, it is this nerve that facilitates improved kidney function, increases blood flow, and thus improves our body's filtration. When the vagus nerve is reached through activation, inflammation in all target organs will be minimized. That nerve even has the ability to control female fertility and orgasms. An inactive or blocked vagus nerve may cause havoc through the mind and body.

Now that we know that the vagus nerve is connected to all the main organs and their proper functioning, we easily conclude that any mental or body or spirit disability, sickness, or disease can be reversed or even cured by triggering and improving the vagus nerve. You can also have positive effects on conditions like anxiety, heart disease, depression and migraine, fibromyalgia, alcohol addiction, digestion, gut problems, memory problems, mood disorders, MS, and even cancer.

DR. JASON ROSENBERG

Vagus nerves can be activated by many recorded forms, such as singing or chanting, music, yoga, meditation, respiratory exercises, general exercise, and just to name a couple. Singing and laughing activate the muscles behind the mouth, stimulating the nerve. Mild exercise and rehabilitation generally increase intestinal fluids, which activate the vagus nerve. Regimented yoga may also improve nerve activation due to movement, but meditation and OM-ing can also enhance vagus nerve function. All this activates the vagus nerve and has one thing in common: tone! Tone!!

Physicians are found to help vibrate the body into a state of health globally and move illness and illnesses such as anxiety, PTSD, migraines, depression, memory problems, chronic pain, sleep problems, and cancer. Dr. Gaynor, director of ontology at the Strang Cornell Cancer Prevention Center in New York and author of Sounds of Healing, said: "You can truly see the disease as a form of disharmony. "We know that the music and the sound have profound effects on the immune system that obviously has much to do with cancer." A study was also conducted in April 2016 involving Alzheimer's patients. Researchers at the University of Toronto, the Wilfrid Laurier University and Hospitals Baycrest Center conducted the study in various phases of the disease and subjected these patients to a 40-hertz sound simulation. With awareness, comprehension, and alertness, they noted "promising" outcomes. " Thalamus and hippocampus, the short-lasting remembering for long-lasting memory, you can't do that. Tomatis claimed to have handled a wide range of diseases effectively by the sound because they were all linked to inner ear issues. Just a few of the conditions he has successfully treated include stuttering, depression, Adhd, concentration problems, and coordination disorders.

VAGUS NERVE

Another study indicates that the Tomatis approach benefits children with ADD. "These studies have shown substantial improvements in Tomatis's processing speed, phonologic understanding, and phonemic decoding efficacy compared with non-Tomatis: the sound group quickly became the most inflamed about alternative healthcare providers. Sound is an outstanding application of traditional medicine to activate the vagus nerve and enhance the body's health and vitality. Do that through Crystal Chakra Singing Bowls and Sound Healing. Clear quartz is called the' Master Healer,' as it can enhance, transform, and relay energy. The impacts in these quartz crystal bowls are intensive on organs, tissues, cells, and on the circulatory, endocrine, and metabolic systems. The crystal pulse is heard by the ear and feels within the body, stimulates the nerve in all the centers of the chakra, which induces harmony and rejuvenation of skin, body and mind.

DR. JASON ROSENBERG

CHAPTER 1

WHAT IS THE VAGUS NERVE?

Did you know that the human body has 12 cranial nerves? Did you know that each "nerve" is actually comprised of two nerves, typically left and right nerve intertwined to make the "one" cranial nerve? And these nerves are the link between your body and the brain? Have you ever wondered how the brain and body "talk" to one another? It is all through these cranial nerves. Some of the nerves are responsible for sharing sensory information, like how something sounds or what it tastes like. This means these nerves need to have the sensory function to interpret the smell of something. But then there are other nerves that "talk" with the muscles and even some glands. These nerves are called "motor functions." And finally, while most have a single function, either sensory or muscle, there are others that operate with both. The Vagus nerve is one such nerve.

To help you understand where a nerve is located, each cranial

VAGUS NERVE

number is assigned a number represented in Roman numerals, for example, I is one, II is two, etc. The Vagus nerve is the tenth nerve and is called CNX, or Cranial Nerve Ten.

In Latin, the word "vagus" is defined as "wandering." When you understand a bit more of the makeup of this nerve, you will realize that this description is pretty accurate. The Vagus nerve is the longest in the human body, and it does a lot of traveling around and through it. Basically, it moves from the base of your skull to your lower torso.

There are two parts to the sensory functions of this particular nerve:

1. Visceral: This is used to describe the "feelings," or sensations, in your body's organs.

2. Somatic: This term is applied to your physical "feelings," or sensations in the muscles and skin of your body.

3. Each part of the sensory function is unique. The somatic function gives information regarding the skin from behind the ears. It also shares this information from the ear canal and various parts of the throat. It is also responsible for the visceral information shared to the brain regarding the majority of your digestive tract, heart, lungs, trachea, esophagus, and larynx. Finally, while it is not the primary "player" in the sensations in your tongue, your Vagus nerve does have a small role in how your tongue's root experiences the sensation of taste.

4. There are three primary motor functions that the Vagus nerve functions with:

5.   Stimulates digestion and the digestive tract. This involves involuntary contractions in the majority of your intestines, stomach, and esophagus to help food move through the system.

6.   Stimulates your heart. The primary goal is to massage the muscles of the heart in an effort to lower your resting heart rate.

7.   Stimulates your mouth. This stimulation includes the soft palate, or the soft area in the back of the roof of your mouth, larynx, and pharynx.

As you can see, this nerve is a fairly powerful player in not just how you feel, but how you experience the world you are living in. It impacts everything from your brain to your digestion, and so much in between. This means if something "goes wrong," it can have dire consequences to your health and well-being. To check to see if it is in working order, many physicians will first begin with your gag reflex. It is often done with a cotton swab, where the doctor "tickles" both sides in your back throat. This causes most people to involuntarily gag. If not, there may be something wrong with this nerve.

Some of the common problems that occur for your Vagus nerve include:

- Nerve damage

- Gastroparesis

- Vasovagal syncope

Nerve Damage

Because of the extreme length and vast scope of this nerve, there can be a variety of symptoms indicating it has been damaged. Most of the time the symptom of Vagus nerve damage depends on the location of the damage. Some of the common symptoms include:

- Stomach acid production is decreased

- Blood pressure is abnormal

- Heart rate is unusual

- Ear pain

- Gag reflux is minimal or lost

- Drinking liquids proves to be a problem

- Wheezy or hoarse voice often

- Loss of voice or challenge speaking

- Vomiting or nausea

- Pain or bloating in the abdomen

Gastroparesis

Gastroparesis is another condition that many experts believe is the result of a damaged Vagus nerve. This concerns the contractions of the digestive tract. When the involuntary contractions are not functioning properly the stomach cannot empty properly. It is a common side effect of vagotomy. This is a procedure that removes some or all of the Vagus nerve. Side effects common to gastroparesis include:

- Blood sugar fluctuations

- Weight loss that is unexplained

- Bloating or bleeding in the abdomen

- Acid reflux

- Feeling full at the beginning of a meal or not having an appetite

- Vomiting or nausea, especially if the vomit contains food that is not digested even hours after eating

What Exactly Are The Causes Of Vagus Nerve Damage?

This particular nerve materials motor nerve impulses on the muscles of the voice box and tongue, receiving sensory desires coming from the organs, ear, and the throat of the chest as well as belly, and also providing visceral nerve impulses to the glands of the throat, abdominal organs, and chest. Female doctor showing healthcare chart to a female patient resting in the hospital bed.

Diabetes

Diabetes is able to result in neuropathy, or maybe nerve damage, to a variety of distinct body parts. A prolonged rise in blood glucose associated with diabetes is able to modify nerve chemistry and harm the blood vessels which support the nerves. In instances where diabetic issues have destroyed the vagus nerve, it is able to result in gastroparesis, a problem whereby the muscles of the stomach, as well as intestine, aren't able to effectively move meals with the gastrointestinal system. Gastroparesis manifests in symptoms including nausea, abdominal bloat, constipation, heartburn, vomiting, stomach spasms, & decreased appetite.

Alcoholism

Chronic alcohol abuse is recognized to damage nerves, a condition called alcohol neuropathy. Alcohol abuse has a dose-related deadly impact on the autonomic nervous system; of that the vagus nerve is a portion. Abstaining from alcohol is able to overturn the harm to the vagus nerve. Infection, as well as Surgical Complications Vagus nerve injury is able to happen following top respiratory viral infections. These infections initially involved signs, for example, cough, runny noses, and nasal congestion. Symptoms that persisted in individuals diagnosed with post-viral vagal neuropathy, throat clearing, included cough, or PVVN, vocal fatigue, and difficulty speaking. The vagus nerve is often damaged during surgery to the small intestine or the stomach. A process known as laparoscopic hemifundoplication, utilized to treat gastric reflux, continues to be connected with vagus nerve injury.

Vasovagal Syncope

During stressful situations, the Vagus nerve can overreact. When this happens it can dramatically drop your blood pressure and heart rate, because it is responsible for stimulating the various muscles in your heart to slow down the heart rate. This sudden drop can lead to fainting. Some common stressful triggers include:

- Standing for long periods of time

- The intense strain on the body, including while trying to have a bowel movement

- Having blood drawn or seeing blood

- The concern of harm to the body

- Extreme heat and overexposure

VAGUS NERVE

CHAPTER 2

UNDERSTANDING POLYVAGAL THEORY: EMOTIONAL SHUTDOWN

The polyvagal hypothesis: New bits of knowledge into versatile responses of the autonomic sensory system

The hypothesis is reliant on gathered information portraying the phylogenetic changes in the vertebrate autonomic sensory system. Its particular spotlight is on the phylogenetic move among reptiles and warm-blooded animals that brought about explicit changes to the vagal pathways managing the heart.

Imagining mind science can be something like envisioning a storm. In spite of the fact that we can envision awful climate, it is hard to envision changing that climate. In any case, Stephen Porges' polyvagal hypothesis gives advocates a valuable image of the sensory system that can direct us in our endeavors Branding-Images_chemistryto help customers.

VAGUS NERVE

Porges' polyvagal hypothesis created out of his investigations with the vagus nerve. The vagus nerve serves the parasympathetic sensory system, which is the quieting part of our sensory system mechanics. The parasympathetic piece of the autonomic sensory system adjusts the thoughtful dynamic part, yet in considerably more nuanced ways than we comprehended before polyvagal hypothesis.

Our three-section sensory system

Before polyvagal hypothesis, our sensory system was envisioned as a two-section hostile framework, with more actuation flagging not so much quieting but rather more quieting flagging less initiation. Polyvagal hypothesis distinguishes a third sort of sensory system reaction that Porges calls the social commitment framework, a fun loving blend of initiation and quieting that works out of one of a kind nerve impact.

The social commitment framework causes us explore connections. Helping our customers move into utilization of their social commitment framework enables them to turn out to be progressively adaptable in their adapting styles.

The two different pieces of our sensory system capacity to assist us with overseeing dangerous circumstances. Most instructors are as of now acquainted with the two safeguard components activated by these two pieces of the sensory system: thoughtful battle or-flight and parasympathetic shutdown, here and there called stop or-swoon. Utilization of our social commitment framework, then again, requires a feeling of security.

Dr. Jason Rosenberg

Polyvagal hypothesis causes us comprehend that the two parts of the vagus nerve quiet the body, however they do as such in various manners. Shutdown, or stop or-swoon, happens through the dorsal part of the vagus nerve. This response can feel like the exhausted muscles and discombobulation of an awful influenza. At the point when the dorsal vagal nerve closes down the body, it can move us into idleness or separation. Notwithstanding influencing the heart and lungs, the dorsal branch influences body working beneath the stomach and is engaged with stomach related problems.

The ventral part of the vagal nerve influences body working over the stomach. This is the branch that serves the social commitment framework. The ventral vagal nerve hoses the body's routinely dynamic state. Picture controlling a pony as you ride it back to the stable. You would keep on pulling back on and discharge the reins in nuanced approaches to guarantee that the pony keeps up a suitable speed. Moreover, the ventral vagal nerve permits initiation in a nuanced way, in this way offering an unexpected quality in comparison to thoughtful enactment.

Ventral vagal discharge into action takes milliseconds, while thoughtful enactment takes seconds and includes different substance responses that are likened to losing the steed's reins. Also, when the battle or-flight concoction responses have started, it can take our bodies 10–20 minutes to come back to our pre-battle/pre-flight state. Ventral vagal discharge into movement doesn't include these sorts of synthetic responses. Along these lines, we can make speedier alterations among actuation and quieting, like what we can do when we utilize the reins to control the steed.

And when you go to a canine park, you will see certain mutts that are apprehensive. They show battle or-flight practices. Different mutts will flag a desire to play. This flagging regularly takes the structure that we people seized for the descending confronting canine posture in yoga. At the point when a pooch gives this sign, it prompts a degree of excitement that can be extreme. In any case, this fun loving vitality has an altogether different soul than the power of battle or-flight practices. This lively soul portrays the social commitment framework. At the point when we experience our condition as sheltered, we work from our social commitment framework.

Injury's impact on sensory system reaction

And when we have uncertain injury from quite a while ago, we may live in a rendition of ceaseless battle or-flight. We might have the option to channel this battle or-flight uneasiness into exercises, for example, cleaning the house, raking the forgets about or working at the rec center, however these exercises will have an unexpected vibe in comparison to they would in the event that they were finished with social commitment science (think "Whistle While You Work").

For some injury survivors, no movement effectively channels their battle or-flight sensations. Subsequently, they feel caught and their bodies shut down. These customers may live in a form of interminable shutdown.

Diminish Levine, a long-lasting companion and partner of Porges, has considered the shutdown reaction through creature perceptions and bodywork with customers. In Waking the Tiger: Healing Trauma, he clarifies that rising up out of shutdown requires a shiver or shake to release suspended battle or-flight vitality. In a perilous circumstance, in the event that we have shut down and an open door for dynamic endurance presents itself, we can wake ourselves up. As instructors, we may perceive this move from shutdown to battle or-trip in a customer's move from gloom into nervousness.

Be that as it may, how might we help our customers move into their social commitment science? And when customers live in a progressively dissociative, discouraged, shutdown way, we should assist them with moving incidentally into battle or-flight. As customers experience battle or-flight power, we should then assist them with finding a feeling of security. At the point when they can detect that they are sheltered, they can move into their social commitment framework.

The body-mindfulness methods that are a piece of intellectual conduct treatment (CBT) and persuasive conduct treatment (DBT) can assist customers with moving out of dissociative, shutdown reactions by urging them to turn out to be increasingly epitomized. At the point when customers are progressively present in their bodies and better ready to take care of flashing solid pressure, they can wake up from a shutdown reaction. As customers initiate out of shutdown and move toward battle or-flight sensations, the idea rebuilding methods that are likewise part of CBT and DBT can instruct customers to assess their wellbeing all the more precisely. Intelligent listening systems can assist customers with feeling an association with their instructors. This makes it workable for these customers to have a sense of security enough to move into social commitment science.

Explicit parts of ventral vagal nerve working

Porges picked the name social commitment framework on the

grounds that the ventral vagal nerve influences the center ear, which sift through foundation clamours to make it simpler to hear the human voice. It additionally influences facial muscles and along these lines the capacity to make open outward appearances. At last, it influences the larynx and in this way vocal tone and vocal designing, helping people make sounds that calm each other.

Polyvagal hypothesis clarifies three unique pieces of our sensory system and their reactions to distressing circumstances. We can perceive any reason why and how we respond to high measures of pressure.

And when polyvagal hypothesis sounds as energizing as watching paint dry, stay, trust me. It's an entrancing clarification of how our body handles passionate pressure, and how we can utilize various treatments it to rework the impact of injury.

Polyvagal theory importance

For advisors, and pop-brain science aficionado the same, understanding polyvagal hypothesis can help with:

- Getting injury and PTSD

- Understanding the move of assault and withdrawal seeing someone

- Seeing how outrageous pressure prompts separation or closing down

- Seeing how to peruse non-verbal communication

DR. JASON ROSENBERG

We like to think about our feelings as ethereal, complex, and hard to sort and recognize.

In all actuality feelings are reactions to an upgrade (interior or outside). Frequently they occur out of our mindfulness, particularly in the event that we are distant, or incongruent, with our internal passionate life.

Our basic want to remain alive is more imperative to our body than even our capacity to consider remaining alive. That is the place polyvagal hypothesis comes in to play.

The sensory system is continually running out of sight, controlling our body capacities so we can consider different things—like what sort of frozen yogurt we'd like to request, or how to get that An in medications school. The whole sensory system works pair with the mind, and can assume control over our enthusiastic experience, regardless of whether we don't need it to.

VAGUS NERVE

Dr. Jason Rosenberg

CHAPTER 3

Vagus Nerve Anatomy And Functions

(VVC) Ventral Vagal Complex: Signaling System for motion, emotion & communication.
(Our Social Engagement System)

(SNS) Sympathetic Nervous System: Mobilization System for Flight or Fight Behaviors.
(Our Aggressive Defense System)

(DVC) Dorsal Vagal Complex: Immobilization System for Conservation Withrawal.
(Our Passive Defense System)

Our Autonomic Nervous System fires muscular tensions triggered by feedback signals from the external & internal world at millisecond speeds below conscious awareness. These muscles tensions fire our Thoughts?

The cranial nerves contain the tactile and engine nerve strands that innervate the head. The cell assemblages of the tactile neurons lie either in receptor organs (e.g., the nose for the smell, or the eye for vision) or inside cranial tangible ganglia, which lie along some cranial nerves only external to the cerebrum. The cranial tactile ganglia are legitimately practically identical to the dorsal root ganglia on the spinal nerves. The cell groups of most cranial engine neurons happen in cranial nerve cores in the ventral dark matter of the cerebrum stem - similarly as cell collections of spinal engine neurons happen in the ventral dim matter

Olfactory Nerve

The Olfactory nerves which subserve the feeling of smell have their cells of the root in the mucous film of the upper and back piece of the nasal hole. They are bipolar tangible cells, the distal parts of which comprise of ciliated procedures that infiltrate the mucous layer in the upper segment of the nasal cavity. The focal procedures of these nerves, around twenty on each side, go through the cribiform plate of the ethmoid cells, the dendrites of which structure brush-like terminals of olfactory glomeruli.

The axons of the mitral cells enter the olfactory nerves of the frontal unresolved issues cerebrum. Posteriorly, the olfactory tract separated into average and horizontal olfactory striae. The average straie goes to the contrary side through the foremost commissure. Filaments in the horizontal striae radiate guarantees to the foremost punctured substance and end in the average and cortical cores of the amygdaloid complex and prepiriform zone. The last speaks to the essential olfactory cortex.

Before assessing olfactory sensations, one must find out that the nasal entries are not blocked. Nearby injuries, for example, unfavorably susceptible rhinitis, polyps, and sinusitis which hinder olfaction must be prohibited. The test substance ought to be non-aggravation and unstable. Crisply ground espresso power, asafoetida, eucalyptus oil or lemon oil are a portion of the basic test substances utilized. Substances like chloroform which may invigorate gustatory end-organs or the fringe endings of the trigeminal nerves in the nasal mucosa as opposed to animating the Olfactory nerves, ought to be stayed away from. Every nostril ought to be tried independently with the other nostril being impeded. The patient ought to be asked to breathed in and recognize the test substance. The view of smell is a higher priority than recognizable proof.

Clutters of Olfaction

- Quantitative: Loss (anosmia), decrease (hyposmia) or expanded keenness (hyperosmia)

- Subjective: Distortion of smell (dysosmia or parosmia)

- Fantasies and pipedreams of smell.

Anosmia happens just if the ailment is two-sided. Hyperosmia is normally an element of masochist patients. Dysosmia or parosmia may happen with neighborhood variations from the norm in the Nose. Olfactory pipedreams and dreams typically propose a mental issue. In any case, they might be related to uncinate seizures where the olfactory experience is brief and joined by an adjustment of awareness and other epileptic wonders.

Optic nerve

Generally, the optical nerve is the association between the eye and the mind. It comprises a gathering of more than one million nerve strands, in spite of the fact that the tissue of the optic nerve is, in reality, more firmly identified with cerebrum tissue than to nerve tissue.

At the point when light enters the eye, it first goes through the cornea. The cornea capacities much as a focal point spread on a camera does. The cornea twists the entering light to guide it towards the understudy and iris. The iris is the hued piece of the eye and the student is the dark hover in the eye.

The student manages the measure of light that enters the eye. The student expands or broadens when there is less encompassing light, permitting all the more light to enter the eye. Alternately, the student diminishes in size when there is a ton of encompassing light, constraining the measure of light that is permitted to enter.

The entering light at that point goes through the perspective of the eye. The focal point helps center the entering light onto the rear of the eye. This territory of the eye is known as the retina, which is a light-touchy layer of nerve cells that changes over the light is gotten to electrical driving forces that are sent to the cerebrum by means of the optic nerve. Curiously, the light and comparing picture is really engaged topsy turvy onto the retina.

The electrical driving forces that are transmitted to the cerebrum by means of the optic nerve are then seen by the mind as a picture. Despite the fact that the picture is at first centered topsy turvy around the retina and transmitted in a similar manner, the cerebrum sees the picture as being straight up.

Since the optical nerve is the channel between the eyes and the cerebrum, any issues related to it can cause issues with vision. Optic nerve hypoplasia is a condition that happens when the optical nerve doesn't grow completely during pregnancy. This can make gentle serious vision hindrance in one of the two eyes.

It isn't known precisely what causes optic nerve hypoplasia and it isn't accepted to be a genetic condition. While there are a few investigations that demonstrate that there might be an association between moms with diabetes, maternal medication and liquor misuse, maternal age under 20 years, and the utilization of hostile to epileptic medications by a mother during pregnancy; inquire about shows that these variables are not factors in a larger part of the instances of optic nerve hypoplasia.

Notwithstanding optic nerve hypoplasia, conditions, for example, sickness, damage, diabetes, hypertension, medication, liquor or tobacco misuse can influence the capacity of the optical nerve to work appropriately, perhaps causing vision disability or even visual impairment.

Oculomotor nerve

One of the hugest nerves that have authority over the majority of the developments identified with the eye, which incorporates the narrowing of the student, is the Oculomotor nerve. It is additionally liable for keeping the eyelids open by innervating the muscles of the levator palpebrae bosses.

VAGUS NERVE

As far as the pecking order, it is gone before by the olfactory and the optic nerve. The oculomotor nerve starts from the third nerve center (discovered ventral to the cerebral reservoir conduit on the focal dim matter) of the unrivaled colliculus. This engine nerve comprises of two separate parts, every one of which has a particular task to carry out. The names of the segments are – substantial engine segment and the instinctive engine segment.

This nerve fuses axons of sort GSE, physical efferent and innervates skeletal muscle of the prevalent, second rate, average and substandard slanted muscles. It innervates all the outside muscles with the exception of the horizontal rectus and the prevalent angled.

This particular engine segment has the capacity of giving four extraocular muscles in the eye alongside the engine filaments to the upper palpebrae superioris. While the visual following is identified with the movement, obsession alludes to the emphasis on a stationary item. For example – a tractor moving continually on the field is visual following and a swallow sitting on a stage is an obsession.

With regards to this specific segment, it participates in overwhelming over some automatic activities of the ciliary muscles and furthermore the constrictor papillae. Other than it additionally has a noteworthy capacity in aiding in settlement and pupillary light reflexes. Settlement can be portrayed as the element that is the capacity of the eye to keep an item's center unblemished in any event when it good ways from the eye. Once more, pupillary eye reflexes are the programmed modifications in the size of the student. Accordingly, it keeps amount and power of the light going into the eye and ensures that it isn't unreasonably glaring for the eye to manage.

Function of Oculomotor nerve

- The oculomotor nerve has somatic and autonomic capacities.

- The oculomotor nerve has three fundamental engine capacities:

- Innervation to the student and focal point (autonomic, parasympathetic)

- Innervation to the upper eyelid (physical)

- Innervation of the eye muscles those take into consideration visual following and look obsession (substantial)

The oculomotor nerve has its engine core in the front piece of the midbrain. The oculomotor nerve broadens anteriorly and separates into predominant and substandard branches, the two of which go through the unrivaled orbital gap into the circle. Axons in the predominant branch innervate the unrivaled rectus (an outward eyeball muscle) and the levator palpebrae superioris (the muscle of the upper eyelid). Axons in the second rate branch supply the average rectus, mediocre rectus, and sub-par sideways muscles - all outward eyeball muscles.

Trochlear nerve

The trochlear nerve, otherwise called the fourth nerve or the fourth cranial nerve, is situated close to the cerebrum and serves the prevalent slanted muscle of the eye. It has a few special highlights in that it contains the least axons of any of the 12 cranial nerves and is the longest. There are two trochlear nerves, one for each eye, and they are found in people as well as in all vertebrates that have jaws.

Trochlear nerve work centers around a solitary muscle that attempts to move the eye. Development made conceivable by the prevalent slanted muscle of the eye incorporates rolling the eye all over and pushing it toward the nose or "intersection" the eyes. The muscle itself appends to the rear of the eyeball, however, a ligament reaching out from it connects to the highest point of the eyeball and applies pressure through a pulley-like structure. This structure clarifies the nerve's name, trochlear, which signifies "pulley" in Latin.

This present nerve's job in controlling developments of the eye is the reason trochlear nerve harm can prompt issues with vision. Specifically, trochlear nerve damage in one eye can hinder that eye's capacity to move in synchronization with the other eye, regularly causing twofold vision. This condition is additionally alluded to as trochlear nerve paralysis. It frequently is analyzed by the patient's inclination to hold their head in a tilted situation so as to mitigate twofold vision.

Alfred Bielschowsky, an ophthalmologist from Germany, built up the head tilt test used to analyze trochlear nerve paralysis. Most of Bielschowsky's work was acted in the main portion of the twentieth century. Despite the fact that tilting of the head can be brought about by different conditions, the Bielschowsky head tilt test stays being used today as an asymptomatic apparatus. Most generally, trochlear nerve paralysis happens because of head injury; however, it additionally has been determined related to have conditions, for example, various sclerosis, diabetes, and atherosclerosis.

Accurate information in regards to recurrence of trochlear

nerve paralysis is dubious, on the grounds that numerous patients essentially make up for the twofold vision through head development. For the individuals who are never again ready to accomplish satisfactory outcomes with pay, treatment, for the most part, includes medical procedure. Careful advancements created during the 1970s have significantly improved treatment choices and viability.

Abducens nerve

This nerve emerges from the lower some portion of the pons on the floor of the fourth ventricle. The nerve rises up out of the cerebrum stem at the pontomedullary intersection. It has the longest intracranial course among all the cranial nerves and lies between the pons and the clivus. It punctures the dura at the dorsum sellae, between the back clinoid and peak of the petrous unresolved issue the enormous sinus, inferomedial to the third nerve. It enters the Orbit through the better Orbital gap than supply the outer (horizontal) rectus muscle.

Facial nerve

Did you realize that the facial nerve controls the muscles on either side of our face and it lets us show our various demeanors from grinning to crying to winking? A similar nerve likewise controls hearing and taste to a degree. This nerve is fundamentally the same as state a phone link, and it contains around 10,000 separate nerve strands. Each fiber conveys electrical driving forces to a specific facial muscle. This motivation conveys data that permits to cry, chuckle, grin, scowl, wink and so forth.

VAGUS NERVE

This nerve additionally conveys driving forces to the tear organs, spit organs and furthermore to the muscle of the stirrup bone in the center ear. So in light of the fact that this nerve performs such huge numbers of various capacities there possibly numerous manifestations if there should arise an occurrence of harm. So a facial nerve issue otherwise called Bells Palsy could bring about loss of motion of the face, jerking, or dryness in the mouth or even the eye, turmoil in the taste and so forth. Any harm to this nerve could cause ruin in any one's life, be it socially or mentally.

5 different ways to beat the indications of facial nerve issues are:

•   To drink warm fluids, for example, tea with cinnamon and ginger to move away the side effects of the infection. A prescribed home cure is to eat garlic with olive oil. To crush the garlic and blend it in with the olive oil and afterward eat it.

•   To keep away from the drain and shield your face from presentation to wind. So consistently secure your face at whatever point you go out.

•   Anti-provocative medications can beat this issue. Steroids are the typical suggestion for conditions influencing the facial nerve. Calming medications may likewise be joined with an antiviral medication called Acyclovir.

•   Lubricating eye drops and treatments can be utilized to shield the eye from contamination and dryness

•   If the facial nerve paralysis is because of a tumor, the typical proposal is medical procedure.

While medicinal treatments can accelerate the physical recuperation of a patient experiencing this issue, close loved ones need to perceive the huge enthusiastic and mental issues goes with this issue. Thusly consistent help from loved ones is a special reward and can enable the patient to recuperate rapidly from facial paralysis issues. Guiding to the two patients and their relatives is likewise prescribed for better treatment and helps in understanding the sickness better.

Glossopharyngeal nerve

Secluded ninth nerve sores are incredibly uncommon. Diphtheria can cause ninth nerve loss of motion.

Glossopharyngeal nerve variations from the norm cause trouble in gulping. There might be diminished sensation to contact or agony over the back tongue, sense of taste, and throat. The muffle reflex is missing in these cases.

Activating exercises for the episodes of agony incorporate gulping, talking, chuckling, hacking, or biting. Slow heartbeat and blacking out have happened with seriously agonizing scenes. At the point when a careful treatment isn't self-evident, hostile to seizure meds, for example, gabapentin, phenytoin, and carbamazepine, and a few antidepressants, similar to amitriptyline, are viable in dealing with the side effects.

VAGUS NERVE

CHAPTER 4

12 Cranial Nerve

Cranial Nerve I

Name: Olfactory

Function: Smell

Nucleus: Does not originate on the brainstem

Origin: Olfactory bulb

Exit from Skull: Foramina in the cribriform plate

Component(s): SVA

Branches: Olfactory filaments

Sensory: Yes

VAGUS NERVE

Function (s): Smell

Location (s): Nose

Special Sense: Yes

Function: The special sense of smell, a SVA nerve – Special Visceral Afferent

Location: Nose

Cranial Nerve II

Name: Optic

Function: Sight

Nucleus: Lateral Geniculate Nucleus

Origin: Thalamus

Exit from Skull: Optic foramen of the optic canal

Component (s): SSA

Branches: None

Sensory: Yes

Function: (s): Vision

Location (s): Retina of the eye

Special Sense: Yes

Function: The special sense of sight

Location: Eye

Cranial Nerve III

Name: Oculomotor

Function: Control of many of the motor muscles of the eye and the constriction of the pupil as well as the accommodation of the eye

Nucleus: Oculomotor nucleus; GSE Nucleus

Nucleus: Edinger-Westphal nucleus; GVE Nucleus

Origin: Midbrain (mesencephalon region)

Exit from Skull: Superior Orbital Fissure

Component (s): GSE and GVE

Branches:

Superior Branch (innervates the superior rectus and the levator palebrae superioris)

Inferior Branch/Division – three branches

(1) Innervates the medial rectus

(2) Innervates the inferior rectus

VAGUS NERVE

(3) Innervates the inferior oblique and the ciliary ganglion

Somatic: Yes

Function: Most of the muscle movements of the eye, GSE – general somatic efferent – originate from the oculomotor nucleus

Muscles Innervated: Muscles of the levator palpebrae superioris, superior rectus, medial rectus, inferior rectus, and inferior oblique muscles – these are extraocular muscles

Autonomic NS: Yes

Innervation: Parasympathetic via the Edinger-Westphal nucleus

Function: Constriction of the pupils via the sphincter pupillae muscle and accommodation via the ciliary muscles

Motor: Yes

Function: Extraocular muscles of the eye

Location (s): Most of the muscles of the eye

Cranial Nerve IV

Name: Trochlear

Function: Depresses, intorts and laterally rotates the eyeball

Nucleus: Trochlear nucleus

Origin: Midbrain

Exit from Skull: Superior Orbital Fissure

Component (s): GSE

Branches: None

Somatic NS: Yes

Muscles Innervated: Superior oblique

Function: Depresses, intorts and laterally rotates the eyeball - also called abduction

Motor: Yes

Function: Depresses, intorts and laterally rotates the eyeball – also called abduction

Location (s): Superior oblique muscle

Cranial Nerve V

Name: Trigeminal

Function: Sensory from the face and the muscles of mastication

Nucleus: Trigeminal nuclei

Origin: Pons

Exit from skull: Superior orbital fissure – V1; GSA component

Exit from skull: Foramen rotundum – V2; GSA component

VAGUS NERVE

Exit from skull: Foramen ovale – V3; SVE component, GSA component

Component (s): GSA - Sensory from the face and SVE - motor muscles of mastication

Branches: V1 – the ophthalmic nerve; V2 – the maxillary nerve; and V3 – the mandibular nerve

Somatic NS: Yes

Function: Sensory to the face – general somatic afferent (GSA).

Location: V1 receives sensory information from the upper portion of the face. V2 receives sensory information from the middle region of the face. V3 supplies sensory information from the lower portion of the face.

Sensory: Yes

Function: Sensory neurons

Location (s): Face

Motor: Yes

Function: Muscles of mastication via V3

Location (s): Muscles of mastication

Special Sense: Yes

Function: Muscles of mastication

Location: Muscles of mastication

Other: There are three main branches of the Trigeminal nerve. They are designated by the following abbreviations: V1 (ophthalmic), V2 (maxillary), and V3 (mandibular). The trigeminal nerve has both sensory and motor components. V1 and V2 contain only sensory information. The V3 nerve is designated in the special visceral efferent (SVE) functional group.

Cranial Nerve VI

Name: Abducens

Function: Abducts the eye

Nucleus: Abducens nucleus

Origin: Pons, junction with medulla

Exit from skull: Superior orbital fissure

Component (s): GSE

Branches: None

Somatic NS: Yes

Function: Abduction of the eye

Muscles Innervated: Lateral rectus muscle

Motor: Yes

Function: Abduction of the eye

Location (s): Lateral rectus Muscle

Cranial Nerve VII

Name: Facial

Function (s): Muscles of facial expression, taste and gland stimulation

Nucleus: Facial motor nucleus - SVE

Nucleus: Superior salivatory nucleus – GVE

Nucleus: Geniculate ganglion - GSA, SVA, GVA

Origin: Junction of the pons and the medulla

Exit from skull: Stylomastoid foramen

Component (s): GSA, GVA, SVA, GVE, and SVE

Branches: Cranial Nerve VII has intracranial and extracranial branches.

Intracranial: The greater petrosal nerve; nerve to stapedius; and the chorda timpani

Extracranial: The posterior auricular; the posterior branch of the digastric muscle as well as the stylohyoid muscle; and the five facial branches as follows: temporal; zygomatic; buccal; marginal mandibular; cervical

DR. JASON ROSENBERG

Somatic NS: Yes

Function: Allows some people to wiggle their ear

Muscles Innervated: Posterior auricular

Autonomic NS: Yes

Innervation: General visceral efferent (GVE) to the submandibular, lacrimal, and sublingual glands as well as the mucosa of the nasal cavity.

Function: Stimulate glandular secretion

Sensory: Yes

Function: Sensation

Location (s): Sensation from the posterior ear (GSA) and sensation from the soft palate and nasal cavity (GVA)

Motor: Yes

Function: Muscles of facial expression – special visceral efferent (SVE) – derived from pharyngeal arches - brachiomotor

Location (s): Most of the muscles of the face

Special Sense: Yes

Function: Taste – special visceral afferent (SVA)

Location: Anterior 2/3 of tongue

VAGUS NERVE

Cranial Nerve VIII

Name: Vestibulocochlear

Function: The Vestibular nerve mediates the sensation of sound, rotation, and gravity which is essential for balance and movement. The vestibular branch carries impulses for equilibrium while the cochlear branch carries impulses for hearing.

Nucleus: Spiral ganglia - hearing

Nucleus: Vestibular ganglion - balance

Origin: Lateral side of the medulla and the lateral end of the trapezoid body of the pons.

Exit from Skull: Interior Auditory Canal

Component (s): SSA

Branches: Two branches - Cochlear nerve; vestibular nerve

Sensory: Yes

Function (s): Hearing and Balance

Location (s): Ear

Special Sense: Yes

Function: Hearing and balance (equilibrium)

Location: Ear

Other: Cranial nerve VIII has two main components and functions. It functions in both the special senses of hearing and balance (equilibrium). There are two main branches of this nerve – the vestibular nerve and the cochlear nerve. The vestibular nerve functions in balance, the cochlear nerve functions in hearing. Hearing and balance are both special senses, and both of these nerve branches contain sensory neurons.

Cranial Nerve IX

Name: Glossopharyngeal

Function: Multiple functions

Nucleus: Solitary nucleus – SVA, GVA

Nucleus: Nucleus ambiguous

Nucleus: Inferior salvatory nucleus - GVE

Nucleus: Spinal nucleus of the trigeminal nerve

Nucleus: Lateral nucleus of vagal trigone

Origin: Upper medulla

Exit from Skull: Jugular Foramen

Component (s): GVA, GVE, SVE, GSA, SVA

Branches: The tympanic nerve; the stylopharyngeal branch, tonsillar branches, nerve to carotid sinus, branches to the posterior tongue, lingual branch, and a communicating branch to the vagus

VAGUS NERVE

and it contributes to the pharyngeal plexus.

Somatic NS: Yes

Innervation: Tympanic membrane, upper pharynx and the posterior one third of the tongue

Function: General Somatic Afferent (GSA) sensory information from the tympanic membrane, upper pharynx and the posterior one third of the tongue

Autonomic NS: Yes

Innervation: General Visceral Efferent (GVE) (neurons from the parotid glad via the Otic Ganglia)

Function: GVE neurons – parasympathetic innervation which cause salivation.

Sensory: Yes

Function (s): General visceral afferent (GVA) sensory information from the carotid sinus and the carotid body

Location (s): Carotid sinus and the carotid body

Motor: Yes

Function (s): SVE innervation - Brachialmotor function

Location (s): Special Visceral Efferent (SVE) nerves to the Stylopharyngeal muscle.

Special Sense: Yes

Function: Taste

Location: This nerve provides the sensation of taste to the posterior one-third of the tongue, as well as the circumvallate papillae.

Other: With cranial nerve X, the glossopharyngeal, is involved in the gag reflex.

Cranial Nerve X

Name: Vagus

Function (s): Multiple functions – parasympathetic innervation, taste,

Nucleus: Dorsal nucleus of vagus nerve – parasympathetic innervation to the intestines and viscera - GVE

Nucleus: Nucleus ambiguous – to the brachial efferent neurons and the parasympathetic neurons to the heart

Nucleus: Solitary nucleus – afferent from taste and afferent from the viscera -

Nucleus: Spinal trigeminal nucleus

Origin: Lateral side of the medulla

Exit from Skull: Jugular Foramen

Component (s): GVE, SVE, SVA, GSA, GVA – general sensory innervation from the thorax and abdominal viscera

VAGUS NERVE

Branches: The auricular nerve; pharyngeal nerve; superior laryngeal nerve; superior cervical cardiac of vagus; inferior cervical cardiac; recurrent laryngeal nerve, branches of the pulmonary plexus; branches of the esophageal plexus; anterior vagal trunk; posterior vagal trunk

Somatic NS: Yes

Innervation: External auditory meatus and the tympanic membrane

Function: Sensory information

Autonomic NS: Yes

Innervation: Pharynx, larynx, organs of the neck, thorax and abdomen

Function: Parasympathetic innervation to the glands of the mucous membranes of the pharynx, larynx, organs in the neck, thorax, and abdomen

Sensory: Yes

Location (s): Taste to the epiglottis (SVA), Sensation from the external auditory meatus and tympanic membrane – general somatic afferent (GSA), GVA – from the thoracic and abdominal visceral including the aortic arch and aortic body

Motor: Yes

Location (s): Muscles of the pharynx and larynx (SVE)

Special Sense: Yes

Function: Taste to the epiglottis of the tongue – special visceral afferent (SVA) and motor innervation to muscles of the pharynx and larynx – special visceral efferent (SVE)

Location: The tongue, the pharynx and the larynx

Other: With cranial nerve IX, the vagus, is involved in the gag reflex.

Cranial Nerve XI

Name: Spinal Accessory

Function: Motor neurons

Nucleus: Spinal accessory

Origin: Cranium and upper spinal cord

Exit from Skull: Jugular foramen

Component (s): SVE

Branches: None

Motor: Yes

Function (s): Motor function of the sternocleidomastoid and the trapezius

Location (s): Sternocleidomastoid and the trapezius

Special Sense: Yes

VAGUS NERVE

Function: Muscles arising from the pharyngeal arches – special visceral afferent

Location: Sternocleidomastoid and the trapezius

Other: Cranial nerve XI is the only cranial nerve that originates in the spinal cord, it then ascends into the cranial space, later it exits the cranium through the jugular foramen

Cranial Nerve XII

Name: Hypoglossal

Function: Motor muscles of the tongue; speech, formation of food bolus – manipulating food in the mouth, swallowing

Nucleus: Hypoglossal nucleus

Origin: Medulla oblongata

Exit from Skull: Hypoglossal Canal

Component (s): GSE

Branches: None

Somatic NS: Yes

Function: Motor muscles of the tongue; speech, formation of food bolus – manipulating food in the mouth, swallowing

Muscles Innervated: Genioglossus, geniohyoid, hyoglossus, styloglossus, thyrohyoid

Dr. Jason Rosenberg

Motor: Yes

Function: Motor muscles of the tongue; speech, formation of food bolus – manipulating food in the mouth, swallowing

Location (s): Muscles of the tongue

VAGUS NERVE

CHAPTER 5

FUNCTIONS OF THE VAGUS NERVE

We would like to further underscore the importance of taking proper care of the nervous system thereby ensuring proper functioning of the vagus nerve and associated biological systems.

Main functions of the vagus nerve

The vagus nerve is one large highway that conducts the flow of information from the biological systems that it controls up to the CNS. This is the main raison d'etre of the vagus nerve. In a manner of speaking, the vagus nerve is like a central command post in which the information comes and goes. Consequently, the vagus nerve provides the CNS with all of the data it needs to keep the body alive.

Let's assume that the vagus nerve simply stops working for whatever reason. In such a situation, the person would simply die. How so?

VAGUS NERVE

If the vagus nerve stops sending information to the CNS, the CNS may conclude that the heart and lungs have stopped functioning. Therefore, the brain may have no choice but to begin shutting down other organ systems as well. This type of response may lead doctors to place a patient on life support.

This example highlights the importance that the vagus nerve has on the body's overall ability to sustain life. Now, let's assume that the vagus nerve is functioning properly, but there is some kind of damage to one of the organ systems. In that case, the vagus nerve relays the data on the damage to the organ system back up to the CNS. The brain then sends back the information through the vagus nerve and adjusts accordingly. For instance, if one lung is severely damaged, the brain may choose to shut down that lung and shift all of the breathing functions to the other healthy lung. This is enough to keep the body alive though not necessarily at peak performance.

In addition, the vagus nerve is the main command post for the digestive system. This is a crucial function to consider since the digestive system provides the body with the nutrition it needs to repair itself, fuel movement and keep cells running along. Hence, the digestive system needs close attention. This causal link between the digestive system and the CNS explains why folks who have undergone a traumatic experience often experience digestive distress. When the nervous system suffers a significant jolt, it is not uncommon to see that it has serious repercussions on the entire network controlled by the vagus nerve.

So, let's move on and take a deeper look at the specific functions that are associated with the vagus nerve.

The Visceral Somatic Function

Given the fact that the vagus nerve is part of the Autonomic Nervous System (ANS), it is inextricably linked to the entire body. Think of it as a main highway that receives traffic from all over the region even if the majority of motorists don't actually plan to stay in that particular area. In a way, the main traffic is just passing through.

Based on that premise, any disruption in the flow of traffic in that area may lead to disruption in the flow of traffic in other seemingly unrelated areas. The same goes for the nervous system and biological functions.

When we refer to a somatic function, we are talking about the reaction that comes as a result of the stimuli in the environment surrounding an organism. In this case, the human body is the organism immersed in a given environment.

As such, the somatic function that the vagus nerve plays is one of constant monitoring and regulation. Think of it as one large pressure valve that looks to regulate the build-up within a large engine. If too much pressure builds up, then the engine may explode. The same goes for the nervous system.

With that in mind, there is one interesting bit of good news... if we could call it that. The body is adept at adjusting to its environment. So, if the individual finds themselves consistently inundated by stressful situations, there is the possibility that the body will become adjusted to such levels of stress. In a way, it creates a "new normal".

An example of this attitude can be seen in the so-called "adrenaline junkies". These people become addicted to extreme sports due to the exhilaration that they get from engaging in a dangerous activity. However, they consistently need to up the ante since their nervous system constantly adjusts to the level of danger in each activity. So, in order to get the same rush, they need to overload their nervous system more and more. Otherwise, they may not find the same amount of enjoyment in the same activities.

As far as the visceral function is concerned, the vagus nerve is constantly tracking the performance of the body's internal organ systems. As a matter of fact, it is designed with a number of automatic switches that are intended to protect the body from grievous damage. Think of these switches like circuit breakers in an electrical system. When the system is overloaded by the electrical current, the circuit breaker is tripped thereby protecting the entire system. If no such breaker existed, the wiring would overheat potentially causing a fire.

The vagus nerve has built-in parameters that prevent the body from overexerting itself to the point where permanent damage is done to organs. Consider this situation:

A person who has been working non-stop for a week may find that after going on little to no sleep, they simply crash and sleep for an extended period of time. This reaction is triggered in the nervous system in order to prevent the heart from literally burning out. This is why drug consumption, the kind that disrupts the nervous system, making it prone for individuals to suffer from cardiac arrest. Since the substance wreaks havoc with the PNS natural regulation mechanisms, the body keeps going until it eventually shuts down.

A good example of this can be seen in modern cars. The car's computer shuts the engine down when it diagnoses a potentially serious problem in the engine. The car's control computer module shuts off the flow of gas, for example, in order to keep the engine from completely failing. The car will restart once the issue has been corrected.

So, just like a car's control module, the vagus nerve serves as the body's main regulation unit. This protects the body's vital organs from failing altogether at which point death would ensue. This is why optimal performance from the vagus nerve is essential to ensuring the body's overall optimal performance.

The Physical Motor Function

Since the vagus nerve is part of the overall ANS, it is also connected to the body's peripheral nervous system which controls the movement of limbs. As such, the vagus nerve is involved in the motor functions of the body.

Now, the vagus nerve itself does not regulate movement, but it does regulate the biological functions that aid movement. The following example will illustrate this point.

When a person engages in physical activity, the CNS broadcasts the necessary signals to the limbs for movement, be it running, swimming, and so on. However, the heart is also responsible for supply blood to the muscles while the lungs need to provide oxygen. Furthermore, there is an increased metabolic response as the body needs to create the energy it requires to sustain the level of physical activity. If the activity exceeds the heart's capacity to pump blood and the lungs' ability to provide oxygen, then the individual may simply get tired and stop moving.

This example highlights how important the vagus nerve is when taking movement into account. High-performance athletes have trained not only for their sport, but also develop stamina. Now, you may have heard of this term, yet it is generally associated to endurance, that is, sustaining physical activity over longer periods of time. But the fact of the matter is that stamina is the body's ability to provide the elements the body needs to sustain prolonged periods of physical activity.

Consequently, the vagus nerve is able to recognize these increased levels of physical activity and make the necessary adjustments so that muscles get the elements they need in order to keep going. It should be noted that the vagus nerve will also recognize when an athlete is becoming overexerted. At which point, the athlete may feel like they can't go on anymore. This is the body's protective measures that keep it from causing serious damage.

This last point illustrates the importance of keeping a balanced nervous system so that the vagus nerve can perform its functions appropriately thereby allowing the body's organ systems to provide the elements that the body requires.

Essential biological functions

These functions are what basically keeps the body alive. After all, if your heart stops breathing, then chances are you are not going to make it.

With that in mind, it is important to note that when the vagus nerve is not functioning at 100%, that is, when there is some kind of disruption, the essential biological systems may begin to go haywire. In some cases, it might be a slow and progressive disruption while in other cases it may be a sudden and shocking disruption.

Let's consider two possible scenarios:

An individual who has been working a stressful job begins to feel the effects of chronic stress over months or even years of accumulated stress. Suddenly, they may develop cardiac conditions, anxiety or even chronic digestive disorders. Yet, the progression of these conditions was so subtle that the person didn't really feel much of a difference.

On the flip side, there is a person who underwent a major traumatic incident, for instance, the loss of a loved one. The stress caused by the sudden loss of a dear person may cause a sudden overload to the nervous system. This sudden overload may lead to the onset of any of the aforementioned conditions. This may prompt swift intervention by medical professionals in order to address the onset of the symptoms the person is experiencing.

In either case, the vagus nerve can come under attack. At this point, there is a serious need for treatment which can correct the imbalances in the nervous system thus promoting recovery from the overwhelming effects on the nervous system. In fact, you may be surprised that some of the most common conditions that you may be familiar with can be addressed by balancing out the vagus nerve's functions.

VAGUS NERVE

CHAPTER 6

ADVANTAGES AND TRUTH ABOUT VAGUS NERVE

1. Vagus nerve averts inflammations.

Quantity of inflammation following illness or injury is ordinary. Vagus nerve works a huge system of fibers clad just like spies in your organs. If it receives a sign for inflammation existence of cytokines or a chemical called as tumor necrosis factor --it alarms the brain and pulls out anti-inflammatory receptors that modulate the body's immune reaction.

2. It makes it possible to make memories.

Stimulating their vagus nerves augments the memory. This activity distributed the neurotransmitter norepinephrine to the amygdala, which merged memories. Associated studies have been performed in humans, indicating promising treatments for ailments, including Alzheimer's disease.

VAGUS NERVE

3. It makes it possible to breathe.

Even the neurotransmitter acetylcholine, elicited from the vagus nerve, which advises your lungs. It is one reason why Botox--frequently used cosmetically--may be potentially harmful, since it disrupts your acetylcholine creation. It's possible, however, to also excite your vagus nerve by performing abdominal breathing or holding your breath for four to eight counts.

4. It is intimately involved with your own heart.

The vagus nerve is responsible for controlling the heartbeat via electric impulses to technical muscle tissues --that the heart's natural pacemaker--at the right atrium, in which acetylcholine release slows down the heartbeat.

By measuring the period between your personal heartbeats, then mimicked this on a graph with time, and physicians can decide your heart rate variability, or HRV. This information can provide clues regarding the durability of your own heart and vagus nerve-stimulation.

5. It starts your system's comfort response.

Whenever your ever-vigilant sympathetic Nervous system pops up the flight or fight responses--massaging the stress hormone adrenaline and cortisol in your own body –that's when the vagus do not tells the human system to chill out by releasing acetylcholine. The vagus nerve's tendrils stretch to a lot of organs, behaving like fiber-optic wires that send directions to release proteins and enzymes such as prolactin, vasopressin, and oxytocin, which calm down you. Individuals with a more powerful vagus reaction might be more inclined to recover more rapidly following anxiety, trauma, or disease.

6. It contrasts between your stomach and your brain.

Your gut employs the vagus nerve like a Walkie-talkie to inform your brain how you are feeling through electrical impulses known as "action potentials." Your gut feelings are extremely real.

7. Overstimulation of the Vagus Nerve is the usual cause of fainting.

Should you shake or get queasy at the sight of blood or while obtaining a flu shot you are not weak. You are experiencing "vagal syncope." Your entire body, reacts to pressure, overstimulates the vagus nerve, thus causing the blood pressure and heart rate to fall. During intense syncope, blood circulation is limited to the brain, and you lose consciousness. But the majority of the time you simply need to lie or sit down for the symptoms to subside.

8. The electrical stimulation of the Vagus nerve decreases inflammation and might inhibit it completely.

Neurosurgeon Kevin Tracey was that the first to demonstrate that stimulating the vagus nerve can considerably reduce inflammation. Outcomes on rats were successful; he replicated the experimentation in people with magnificent results. The development of enhancements to stimulate the vagus nerve through digital implants revealed a radical reduction, and sometimes even remission, in rheumatoid arthritis--that has no known treatment and is frequently treated together with the poisonous medications --hemorrhagic shock, along with other equally severe inflammatory syndromes.

9. Vagus nerve stimulation has brought in a new area of medicine.

Spurred on from the achievement of vagal nerve stimulation to treat swelling and epilepsy, a cosmopolitan area of health study, called bioelectronics, could be the future of medication. Using implants which provide electrical impulses to various body components, scientists and physicians hope to take care of illness with fewer drugs and fewer unwanted side effects.

VNS is not a cure, and also the complete elimination of infection is rare. But a lot of men and women who experience VNS undergo a substantial (greater than 50 percent) decrease in the incidence of seizures, in addition to a decline in seizure severity. This can considerably enhance the standard of life for those who have epilepsy.

Depression And Stress: How to Recognize and Treat Coexisting Infection

Anxiety and depression can happen at the exact identical moment. In reality, it's been projected that 45 percentage of individuals with one psychological health state meet the standards for a couple of disorders.

Though each state has its very own triggers, they can share similar symptoms and remedies. Keep reading to find out, including getting strategies for direction and what to anticipate from a medical investigation.

What Are The Signs Of Each Illness?

Some signs of depression and anxiety overlap, like difficulties with sleep, irritability, depression, and trouble concentrating. However there are many important differences which help differentiate between both.

Depression

Feeling down, sad, or angry is normal. It may be about feeling that way for many days or months on end.

Physical signs and behavioral changes brought on by depression comprise:

- Diminished energy, chronic fatigue, or feeling lethargic frequently

- Trouble concentrating, making decisions, or remembering

- Pain, aches, aches, or gastrointestinal troubles with no obvious cause

- Fluctuations in appetite or weight

- Trouble sleeping, waking early, or oversleeping

Emotional Signs of depression comprise:

- Reduction of interest or some more finding enjoyment in hobbies or activities

- Persistent feelings of sadness, anxiety, or bitterness

- Feeling hopeless or pessimistic

- Anger, irritability, or restlessness

- Feeling guilty or undergoing feelings of worthlessness or feedback

- Ideas of suicide or death

- Suicide efforts

- Stress

Stress, or anxiety and nervousness, can happen to anybody from time to time. It is not uncommon to experience stress prior to a huge event or a significant choice.

However, chronic stress could be painful and lead to irrational ideas and fears that interfere with your everyday life.

Physical signs and behavioral changes brought on by generalized anxiety disorder comprise:

- Feeling exhausted easily

- Trouble concentrating or remembering

- Muscle strain

- Fast heartrate

- Jagged teeth

- Sleep problems, such as difficulties falling asleep and

restless, unsatisfying sleep

Psychological symptoms of stress comprise:

- Restlessness, irritability, or feeling on edge

- Trouble commanding fear or anxiety

- Fear

A Self-Help Test Might Help You Determine The Indications

You know what is normal for you. If you end up experiencing feelings or behaviors that are not typical or when something sounds off, this may be an indication you will want to seek out assistance from a health care provider. It is always preferable to chat about what you are experiencing and feeling in order that treatment can start early if it's needed.

With that said, some online self-diagnosis evaluations are readily available to assist you understand what could be occurring. These evaluations, while useful, are not a replacement for an expert diagnosis from your physician. They cannot take different ailments which could be impacting your wellbeing into consideration, either.

Popular self-help evaluations for stress and depression comprise:

- Depression test and stress evaluation

- Depression evaluation

- Stress evaluation

The Way To Handle Your Symptoms

VAGUS NERVE

Besides a proper therapy strategy from your physician, these plans might assist you in finding relief from your symptoms. It is very important to understand, however, these hints might not work for everybody, and they might not work every time.

The objective of treating depression and stress is to produce several treatment choices which may all work together to aid, to an extent, whenever you want to use them.

1.	Allow yourself to feel that which you are feeling -- and also understand that it is not your fault

Anxiety and anxiety disorders are all medical ailments. They are not the consequence of weakness or failure. What you believe is the end result of inherent causes and causes; it isn't the consequence of something that you did or did not do.

2.	Do something that you have control over, such as making your bed or carrying out the garbage

At the moment, regaining a little power or control can help you deal with overwhelming symptoms. Accomplish a job you're able to handle, like neatly restacking publications or sorting out your recycling. Do something to give yourself a feeling of achievement and energy.

3.	You May also create a morning, day, or daily regular activity

Regular activity is occasionally useful for individuals with depression and anxiety. This gives structure and a feeling of control. Additionally, it lets you make space in your daily life for self-care techniques which can enable you to control the symptoms.

4.   Do your best to adhere to some sleep program

Aim to get seven to eight hours per night. Less or more than this will complicate symptoms of conditions. Insufficient or inadequate sleep may cause issues with your own cardiovascular, endocrine, immune, and nervous disorders.

5.   Attempt to eat something healthy, Like an apple or some nuts, at least one time each day

If you are feeling miserable or stressed, you might reach for soothing foods such as sweets and pasta to relieve some of the strain. Nonetheless, these foods offer little nutrition. Try to help nourish your using vegetables, fruits, lean meats, and whole grains.

6.   If you are up for it, then go for a walk round the block

Exercise may be an effective remedy for depression since it is a natural mood booster and also releases hormones that are feel-good. But for many individuals, a gym may cause anxiety and anxiety. If that is true for you, start looking for more natural approaches to use, like walking around your area or searching for an Internet exercise movie you can perform in the home.

7.   Do something which you know brings you relaxation, like seeing a favorite film or writing in a journal

Give yourself time to focus on you along with the things you prefer. Down time is a good way to allow your body to rest, and it may distract your brain with things which bring you an increase in energy.

8.   In case you haven't left the home in some time, look at

doing whatever you find calming, such as getting your nails done or obtaining a massage.

Relaxation techniques may enhance your wellbeing and might lessen symptoms of depression and nervousness. Find an action that feels appropriate for you personally and you can exercise frequently, for example:

Yoga

Meditation

Breathing exercises

Massage

9. Reach out to someone you are comfortable speaking to and speak about anything you want, like how you are feeling or talk about anything you watched on Twitter.

Strong relationships are just one of the best approaches that will assist you in feeling much better. Connecting using a buddy or relative could offer a natural boost and permit you to locate a trusted supply of encouragement and support.

11 Tactics To Reduce Vagus Nerve Work For Improved Gut & Mental Health

1. Try deep breathing or meditation (or even both!) .

Deep breathing is among the very simple yet powerful tactics to stimulate the vagus nerve. Whenever your brain is a couple of counts more than your inhale, then the vagus nerve sends a signal to your brain to turn on your nervous system. Try this workout: Sit for 2 seconds in, and then four seconds outside, using a 1 count pause near the peak of the inhale plus a 1 count pause at the base of the exhale. Numerous studies also encourage the ability of meditation to enhance sleep, pain, hunger, stress, and digestive function using an immediate impact upon vagal tone.

2. Go to a yoga course.

Engaging in regular mild exercise like yoga increases gastric motility— the contractions of the adrenal muscle are essential for the movement of food through the gastrointestinal tract--so it does so through stimulating the vagus nerve.

3. Simply take a cold shower.

Look at finishing your bathing with a one-minute burst of chilly water, and do not be scared to go out for a walk if it is chilly. Studies indicate that intense cold exposure triggers the vagus nerve-stimulation, in addition to different neurons around the vagus nerve pathway, also resulting in a change toward autonomic nervous system action.

4. Eat foods full of tryptophan.

Dietary Tryptophan is metabolized in the intestine and might assist the astrocytes--cells in the brain and spinal cord control inflammation, which might enhance communication From the gut into the brain through the vagal messenger walkway. These meals include spinach, seeds, peas, and poultry.

5. Keep a wholesome weight.

Gut and stomach inflammation may disrupt vagal action and negatively alter the link between the brain and the GI tract. Therefore, if you are obese, your very best choice is to embrace sustainable practices which will cause long-term weight reduction. My information: Move your system every day and concentrate on consuming a diet high in many different fruits and vegetables, together with seeds, nuts, and legumes like the Mediterranean diet.

6. Ensure that you poop every day.

Eat loads of fiber-rich foods daily (target for 25-plus g), and keep regular sleep routines to enable your body to move to a daily rhythm. Healthful removal of waste ensures significantly less stagnation of inflammatory foods residues from the colon, and also a much less hospitable environment for undesirable organisms which could impair communication between the gut and brain.

7. Nix sugar in your diet plan.

Excessive sugar causes chronic inflammation but also soothes cell feedback loops along with other signaling pathways, and also inflammation of the GI tract disease lining allows germs to perpetuate inflammatory signals into the brain.

8. Pop a probiotic.

Along with bettering your ingestion of sugar to boost a wholesome gut and keep optimum gut-brain signaling, look at adding fermented foods along with a probiotic to a daily diet. Research proves that gut bacteria can in fact trigger the vagus nerve. In 1 study, mice which were given the probiotic Lactobacillus rhamnosus experienced improved GABA creation and a decrease in anxiety, depression, and stress. But this favorable effect didn't happen among mice whose vagus nerve was eliminated.

9. Should you consume plenty of creature protein, scale.

Red eggs and meat include choline, which may be helpful for you, but if consumed in excess will be switched into trimethylamine N-oxide (TMAO), a chemical that's been related to cardiovascular and inflammation troubles. Decreased consumption of those foods can reduce inflammation and permit the vagus nerve to regulate cerebral and sympathetic vitals like blood pressure and heartbeat.

10. Contemplate intermittent fasting.

Some research suggests that fasting and dietary restriction may trigger the vagus nerve. And provided that fasting's host of additional advantages --from enhanced cognitive functioning for weight loss to decreased inflammation it could possibly be well worth a try. The very best part: The fasting window does not have to be that much time to reap several fantastic advantages.

11. Belt out your favorite song.

Research also shows that singing includes a biologically calming effect, that has all to do with all the vagus nerve. Go ahead, sing with the radio if you are in the car --or even better, when you're taking a cold shower!

Panic Attacks and Anxiety

As with depression, disorders linked to anxiety and panic attacks often have a stress-related correlation.

Struggling with issues that cause you to feel ill-at-ease and have you experience extreme stress and that can manifest in fear and nervousness for reasons that are not clear.

Panic attacks and anxiety attacks are usually thought to be interchangeable. However, they are very different. Although they have some similar symptoms, there are differences that are distinct in how they manifest, how they are triggered, the length of time they last and how each is treated.

It is important to understand how different each attack is so your symptoms can be reported to your physician accurately. Their treatment is different.

The onset of an anxiety attack is different, whereas it is a gradual escalation of emotions. It is usually caused by a particular situation that can be targeted as the cause of the attack.

Symptoms of an anxiety attack before it occurs can be the feelings of worry, uneasiness, fearfulness or distress. These feelings usually begin before the actual attack and continue after the attack ends.

An anxiety attack can last longer than 10 minutes. If a certain situation is occurring that has caused the attack, the anxiety will continue until the situation changes or ends.

Panic attacks, on the other hand, come on instantaneously and spontaneously. This attack is instant. There is no gradual escalation, it just comes at any time, no matter what the situation. There is usually no identifiable reason why the attack occurred.

While you're experiencing the attack, you will experience crippling fear, as well as the fear of losing control. You also have a feeling of disassociation from your surroundings, known as derealization. You may also experience a detachment from yourself, known as depersonalization.

Panic attacks last, on average, approximately 10 minutes. After the attack ends, the symptoms dispel after the attack ends (Boring-Bray, 2018).

Physical symptoms for both attacks:

- Nausea

- Lightheadedness and/or dizziness

- Pains in the chest

- Difficulty in breathing

- Sweating

- Throat tightening or choking sensation

- Physical shaking or trembling

- Tingling or numbness

- Headache

VAGUS NERVE

If the panic attacks or uncontrolled anxiety attacks persist or accelerate in their occurrence, meeting with a psychologist or a counselor may be a step in the positive direction of dealing with the source of the issue.

DR. JASON ROSENBERG

CHAPTER 7

PTSD

PTSD, or post-traumatic stress disorder, has gained considerable attention in recent years due to its occurrence among military veterans, especially those returning from the long, ongoing conflicts in the Middle East. These traumatized individuals may have experienced severe physical injuries, but in many cases, however, their injuries are psychological, resulting from their overwhelming reactions to their battlefield experiences. In earlier wars, mentally traumatized veterans were said to be suffering from shell shock, the result of seeing and feeling the consequences of war. We now recognize this condition as PTSD.

Typical symptoms of PTSD include flashbacks of the traumatic event or the inability to stop thinking about it obsessively, anxiety, depression, sleeplessness and recurring nightmares. Beyond the discomforts of experiencing PTSD, it is now known that it can lead to suicidal thoughts and suicidal behavior. In many cases, PTSD can lead to continuing deep depression and anxiety, as well as eating disorders, and substance abuse, notably drugs and alcohol.

Apart from veterans, people in all walks of life may have had terrifying, traumatic experiences, either themselves or as witnesses, that trigger PTSD, like an automobile accident, sexual or other physical assault, a serious fall at home, or loss of a loved one. Any of these extremely distressing experiences may initiate the PTSD response. Previously, victims of PTSD may have been told to shape up or get over it, but today, PTSD is a recognized, serious psychological condition requiring professional assistance to resolve. It may affect children as well as adults.

Based on the Polyvagal Theory, it is now believed by many psychologists that PTSD has its roots in the dorsal vagal response of the parasympathetic nervous system. This is the primitive freezing, or shutting down mechanism that is triggered when the person or animal faces an insurmountable or overwhelming immediate threat. When this dorsal vagal response is initiated, it can cause immobility, speechlessness, fainting and even severe shock. PTSD appears to be an ongoing form of dorsal vagal reaction.

The Three-Part Brain

The human brain, with its complexity of 100 billion or so neurons and perhaps 100 trillion neural connections, is generally known to be organized into two hemispheres, the left, recognized for controlling rational, logical, organizational thoughts, and the right, associated with creative, imaginative and unstructured thinking. We also know that the functioning nervous system is comprised of the brain, spinal cord, and between them, the brainstem.

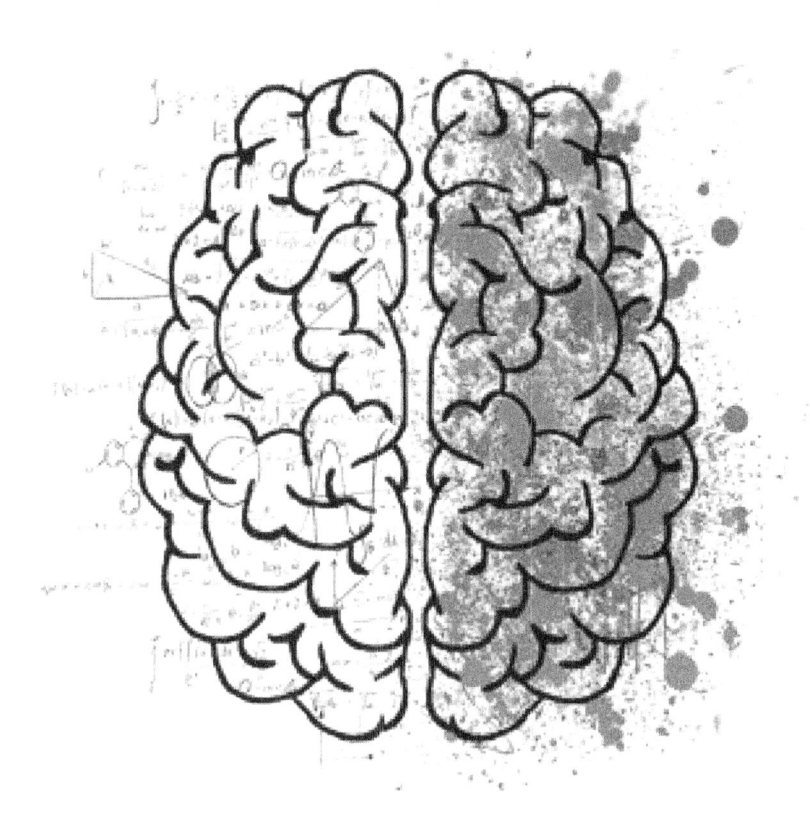

The brain is where all the conscious and unconscious action takes place, from managing our cardiovascular, respiratory and digestive functions to feelings, senses and sensations, and embracing all thought, memory and decision-making.

The spinal cord is the central cable that receives all nerve impulses from the extremities and forwards these impulses to the brain, and returns the brain's reactions to the impulses with the appropriate reaction.

The brainstem is where 10 of the 12 cranial nerves originate and extend to the organs and other key areas, including number 10, the longest, most diverse neuron, the vagus nerve.

VAGUS NERVE

But we know today that the evolution of the human brain has been built upon a sequential three-part structure, beginning with the earliest, most primitive part, called the reptilian brain, then continuing to evolve an early old or paleomammalian brain, and concluding with a more sophisticated new or neo-mammalian brain. This concept of a three-part evolution-driven brain structure was identified first in the 1960's by a neuroscientist, Dr. Paul MaLean, who called it the triune brain, and postulated that these three parts of the brain still struggle to coexist. Each part has specific functions to perform:

The early, reptilian brain, is responsible for basic, involuntary reflex actions, including reproduction urges, arousal to a range of stimuli and maintaining a balanced, normal state, or homeostasis. It can be considered a fundamental survival mechanism. One of its continuing characteristics is compulsiveness.

The old-mammalian, or paleomammalian brain, is positioned to surround the reptilian brain, it manages emotions, learning and memory functions. It enabled early mammals to remember and act upon favorable and unfavorable experiences, for example.

The new-mammalian, or neo-mammalian brain is responsible for conscious thought and self-awareness, and is positioned atop the two early brain parts. All of our reasoning, decision-making and rationalizations occur here.

But one may ask if we really evolved from reptiles? The concept of our brains evolving from reptiles comes as a surprise. We understand that we evolved from mammals, since we ourselves are mammals. Okay, but reptiles? Over the long course of evolution, the earliest mammals evolved from, yes, reptiles, and not from the dinosaurs that became extinct 66 million years ago, or the dinosaurs that grew feathers and evolved into birds. Our reptilian ancestors were small, and obviously smarter than the large dinosaurs, which gave them an edge in natural selection. They had strong survival skills built into their small but highly functional reptilian brains, and some of these hardy reptiles evolved into small mammals. In their turn, these early mammals evolved more complex brains, the paleomammalian brain, with its added values of learning, memory and emotion. Still later, as mammals further evolved as primates, the third neo-mammalian brain component developed, giving Homo Sapiens the ability to think consciously and with increasing complexity.

The three parts of our current triune brain correspond, approximately, to the brainstem and cerebellum (reptilian), limbic brain, which includes the hippocampus, amygdala, and hypothalamus (paleomammalian) and the neocortex (neo-mammalian). Because the reptilian-originated brainstem reacts completely unconsciously and immediately for survival, historically, it tends to dominate in many situations, when the brain perceives a danger or other need for prompt action. The conflict between the purely instinctive reptilian brain and the two more advanced components is considered by some to be represented by Freud's ongoing battles between the conscious and the subconscious.

These aspects include the two-hemisphere structure, vertical networks connecting the layers and departments of the brain, and a near infinite number of interacting neurons, as well as variations in brain structure due to gender, genetic and environmental influences.

In recent times, the precise sequential evolution and functioning of the triune brain, and its exclusivity among humans have been questioned by some animal behaviorists, since complex brains have developed among non-mammal species, including certain birds. Also, new studies demonstrate that in humans, the prefrontal cortex performs complex functions that are apart from the functions of the neocortex.

Post-Traumatic Brain Reeducation

Separate from the psychological disorders associated with PTSD, there are physical brain injuries resulting in serious trauma. About 10 million people worldwide suffer traumatic brain injury (TBI) each year, and many cases are fatal, and most who survive the injury experience some degree of cognitive impairment. These trauma may occur in any number of circumstances, including vehicular accidents, sports injuries, falls inside and outside the home, acts of conflict or violence, even being struck by falling objects.

There are a range of treatments to reverse the impairment, and the type and duration of treatment depends on the type and severity of the trauma. Generally, a multidisciplinary set of treatments is required, involving the psychiatric and neurologic medical practices, as well as pharmacotherapy.

Classifying TBI as mild, moderate or severe depends on several key factors: Degree of post-traumatic consciousness, duration of the coma, if experienced by the patient, and the degree and duration of post-traumatic amnesia. Generally, TBI patients whose symptoms continue for one month or more are classified as either moderate or severe, and whose full recovery make takes years, while those showing marked improvement within a few weeks are considered to be mild cases and often return to full cognitive function within two months.

There are a number of impairments to the cognitive functions following TBI. These are the most commonly treated:

- Decreased ability to concentrate

- Impaired attentiveness

- Reduced visual spatial cognizance

- Tendency to be easily distracted

- Memory lapses and impairments

- Loss of executive ability (decision-making)

- Disrupted communications skills

- Judgmental lapses and dysfunctions

Reeducation of TBI patients begins with assessments based on standardized testing protocols, including visual and auditory attentiveness, visual and verbal measurements, language comprehension and understanding, executive function (decisiveness), overall mental and intellectual function and motor function.

Post-traumatic brain reeducation is undertaken primarily through cognitive rehabilitation, which works to increase the injured person's abilities in the processing and interpretation of information, and the overall performance of mental functions. Cognitive rehabilitation is mostly effective in mild or moderate levels of TBI and with persons who have a high level of motivation to succeed in the recovery. The multidisciplinary group that collaborates on brain reeducational therapy may include doctors, speech and language specialists, physical and occupational therapists, among others. However, it is recognized that each patient's treatment will be unique, prescribed and tailored to each individual, based on the specific injuries suffered and resultant trauma.

One important approach that has wide application is attention process training (ATP), which is based on mental skills training, gradually increasing the complexity of the exercises, from simple initially, and subsequently increasing in complexity, forcing the brain to retrain itself. The exercises include selective attention, focused attentiveness, alternating attention, divided attentiveness and sustained attentiveness.

The Parasympathetic Recovery

The Polyvagal Theory links PTSD to one dimension of the parasympathetic nervous system (PNS), the early-evolved dorsal vagal freeze survival mechanism. The dorsal vagal mechanism may protect an animal by allowing it to play dead until the coast is clear, but in a human being, it can lead to inaction, inability to think or speak, or worse, passing out or fainting, shock or even cardiac arrest. With the linking of PTSD to the dorsal vagal mechanism, a previously unrecognized cause may now be open to evaluation and potentially, to alleviate the symptoms of PTSD.

Specifically, the other, more recently evolved PNS response, the calming, relaxing, socially engaging ventral vagal response may be applied to reduce the emotional and physical symptoms of PTSD. Now the methods used to achieve vagal tone and lower heart rates and breathing rates, reactivate the digestive system and induce an all-encompassing state of calm and relaxation may be applied by the individual, easily, every day. The practice of deep, slow breathing, with forceful extension of the diaphragm to tone the vagus nerve, is applicable as part of meditation or Yoga, or simply done without other techniques.

It can also include auricular and facial massage, massage of the vagus nerve as it passes next to the right and left carotid artery in the neck, and cold facial therapy. The practice of mindfulness, or being in the moment, in which all outside thoughts are prevented from intruding, can also be beneficial, as the person concentrates on every external sound, every feeling, every awareness of things in the environment. Vocal stimulation of the vagus nerve can be done easily by singing, gargling, or reciting a mantra while performing mantra and transcendental meditation.

Another application of Polyvagal Theory to treating PTSD is for the individual to recognize that the symptoms of PTSD are biological in nature, caused by the body's primitive instincts and reflexes to protect itself, and that the body can be taught to relax, get over it, rejoin and socially engage with those who are living active, normal lifestyles. This is called somatic awareness, and it trains the individual to become aware of basic bodily functions like heart rate and breathing, and to consciously try to slow them down. The deep breathing exercises may be helpful in achieving a sense of bodily control.

The reduction or elimination of PTSD symptoms can further be achieved by practicing a series of mental exercises called attentional control, a conscious effort to recognize the cues that may trigger PTSD reactions, and gently but firmly cancel them out by acknowledging that there is no danger, nothing to fear, and all is well. This form of body awareness is called cognitive behavior therapy (CBT), and it encourages the individual to be aware that an unneeded fight or flight response is continuing and can be shut down by conscious thought, replacing disturbing thoughts and memories with relaxing, peaceful thoughts. Over time and with practice, the replacement of bad thoughts with positive ones will make the cooling down of the dorsal vagal action-orientation easier.

Reading Body Language

Body language has long been associated with a few popular positions and movements that are believed to be subconscious cues as to a person's true meaning or intentions. For example, having one's arms crossed signals a negative interest in what is being said, or a hand over one's mouth while speaking may be a sign of a lie being told. Unconsciously nodding one's head indicates agreement, a handshake suggests type of character, depending on whether it is firm or weak, and if eye contact is maintained or not. In reality, most of these body language cues are anecdotal and may have some basis, or they may not.

But Polyvagal Theory has shed a new light on body language, on multiple levels, by revealing one's interest in a social engagement, for example, or sending a signal that can trigger social engagement or other interaction in the second person, who may, in turn, respond with their own body language subconsciously. The use of facial expressions to elicit various types of responses is being used to communicate and engage with autistic children, in testimony to the effectiveness of this approach.

Do the popular body language signals really mean anything, or are they, as implied above, merely anecdotal, believed and circulated but without substantiation? A study conducted by UCLA found that only 7% of what is said is actually believed or acknowledged, based only on the words spoken. The tonality of the speaker's voice accounts for 38% of communications, leaving 50% of communications being based on body language, gestures and expressions.

Resistance to what is being said or shown is frequently shown by crossed arms and crossed legs.

A smile is not sincere when it is limited to the mouth, whereas a sincere smile engages more of the face, including crinkling the eyes.

Mirroring or imitating your own body positions is a sign that the other person is in agreement with what you are saying or proposing.

Power positions radiate a sense of command or control. A person who assumes control will tend to stand upright, extend arms and otherwise occupy more space in a room. This type of person is encouraging interaction or possibly engagement.

Eye contact is not always synonymous with engagement or interest because extended or prolonged eye contact may be forced or deliberate, suggesting the person is hiding a true intention.

Discomfort or surprise may cause raised eyebrows. Conversely, a truly interested person will not tend to raise their eyebrows when spoken to, except to acknowledge an exceptionally unusual remark.

Nodding is positive, except when it's exaggerated because too much nodding suggests discomfort with what is being said.

Tension signals stress. A furrowed brow, tightened neck muscles or a clenched jaw may be signs that what is being said is making the person uncomfortable.

Are these findings valid? Many people you may be speaking with, or meet in an interview, may be consciously nodding or smiling or firmly shaking your hand, deliberately trying to make a good impression. You, in turn, might consider your own body language, and try not to send the wrong message.

The Polyvagal Theory And Emotional Stress

Among the more profound conclusions emerging from Dr. Porges' Polyvagal Theory is the linking of the emotional and physical responses we are subject to. Emotional reactions can trigger not one but two physical responses: the well-known defensive call to action of the sympathetic nervous system, and the more primal dorsal vagal response that can freeze and immobilize a person. Physical actions, conversely, like Yoga, meditation, managed breathing and massages can tone the vagus nerve, triggering the calming, relaxing emotions of the parasympathetic nervous system (also called the ventral vagal response), and its enablement of social engagement.

CHAPTER 8

VAGUS NERVE - MENTAL HEALTH AND OTHER HEALTH ISSUES.

The Vagus Nerve and the Phobias

People often hear about or experience others having fear of certain things and that's not necessarily worrisome but when it grows fiercer and intense, it's definitely something to be worried about. The fear from a certain thing, situation or an entity when grows stronger, it is termed as a phobia. Phobias are of so many types and they are all intense whatever kind they are. Also, it's impossible to escape it because it's an unavoidable facet of human life. Hey! Don't bite your nails out of fear now! The vagus nerve has the solution to your problem but prior to jumping in let's find out the biological presence of phobia in a human brain and its types (of course, not all!).

Phobia unlike fear is not a rush of terror that just passes away when the horror movie ends. These are mental disorders that even doctors diagnose in patients. The patients when come in contact with what triggers their phobia either freeze, get a panic attack, forget to breath and face intense distress and in some cases they die too out of a heart attack. Yes, it's that serious! Now, what causes phobia?

It often starts in childhood; it could be acquired from a parent or a family member. Also, there are some events that cause this such as a near death experience involving an object or an entity which then begins to haunt them for a lifetime. It could be a drowning experience where they got lucky and saved in time, it could be a terrifying or a traumatic event involving darkness. It could be anything, there are no specific causes. Now, when the brain witnesses all of that, it stores it somewhere and then replay it in mind after been triggered to do so; that is when the object, situation or an entity they are afraid of appears in front of them. These chemical reactions take place in amygdala which causes the stress to overpower the patient and they feel intense fear surfacing namely their phobia. Now, let's discuss its symptoms which are:

•	The person who has a phobia would experience anxiety when exposed to the object which they fear.

•	They would avoid that certain thing at all cost.

•	They cease to function well when they come face to face with that thing they fear.

•	The patients will also acknowledge how irrational their fear is and how they don't have anything to do with it.

Also, the physical effects bombard the patient which are:

- Dizziness
- Sweating
- Dry mouth
- Pins and needles
- Butterfly in the stomach
- Headache
- Nausea
- Accelerated heartbeat
- Confusion and alienation
- A chocking sensation
- Shivering
- Chills
- Hot flushes
- Abnormal breathing

These are the symptoms also there are signs such as people becoming clingy.

When you notice such things in yourself or people around you, worry not! It can be easily dealt with.

There are many types of phobias, some of them are:

1. Glossophobia: fear of public speaking.

2. Claustrophobia: fear of small places.

3. Aquaphobia: fear of water.

4. BII (Blood, injury and injection) phobia: the name says it all.

5. Tunnel phobia: fear of tunnels.

6. Nyctophobia: fear of the dark.

7. Acrophobia: fear of heights.

8. Zoophobia: fear of animals.

9. Astraphobia: fear of thunder and lighting.

10. Aerophobia: fear of flying.

11. Arachnophobia: fear of spiders.

12. Haphephobia: fear of touching or being touched.

13. Amaxophobia: fear of driving a car.

14. Ataxophobia: fear of untidiness.

15. Atychiophobia: fear of failure.

All these fears have a history etched to them, for instance, people afraid of Haphephobia may have a history of sexual assault. Similarly, people having Acrophobia may have a near death experience involving falling from any height. Just like that, there are certain reasons people develop these phobias and they grow gradually as the people grow. But be delighted! Vagus nerve is there to put an end to your fears and phobias and let you live a quality life. How?

Well, let's check it out!

Our vagus nerve is joined to our brain from one end and the other to all the organs of the body, basically, it is the one that commands the brain to execute orders therefore, when the panic rise and the phobia is triggered, the vagus nerve is stimulated and causes the fight or flight response to emerge. This helps the person get out of the situation quicker by fighting it or flying it. The therapists make use of certain techniques which stimulate the vagus nerve of the people. They let the patients face, deliberately, what they fear and have phobia of. With this exposure, they instruct the patient to take deep breaths which are the vagus nerve stimulators. The therapists also ask the patient to sit back and relax which also, is a vagus nerve stimulator.

So, when the fear begins to wash over the patient, the vagus nerve stimulation process and steps are applied to the them and the doctors even ask them to exercise and consult a friend to let it all loose. This ultimately causes them to relax and strengthen themselves against their phobias.

Told you! It's a lifesaver!

The Vagus Nerve and Trauma

Trauma is an emotional as well as a psychological response to any frightening and a shockingly heart wrenching event. Those events range from accidents to natural disasters and calamities human mind takes time get over or goes in deep shock after witnessing them. These incidents cause people to be overcame by shock and at times, it causes them to go in denial. This often results in profuse sadness after the damaging event such as death of a beloved, a severe injury, a breakup, verbal humiliation or insult at some point of life or any other painful happenings. Trauma depends on the human brain and its capacity to remember every single detail about what the happiness absorbing event that occurred to cause them sleepless nights and panic attacks.

Now, there are three types of traumas that are very common in people, these are the ones that cause distress to strengthen its roots in the hearts of people, let's find out the names of the culprits:

- Complex trauma:

It is a recurring trauma, this occurs in a certain environment and situation. This causes the person to have panic attacks when exposed to a certain object or thing. It keeps growing intense if not treated on time.

- Post-traumatic stress disorder (PTSD):

Many individuals are aware of this trauma that is very popular amongst people of different ages, this occurs after a bone-chilling, heart breaking event. It could be any experience associated with physical harm or any near death experience. People suffering from

PTSD are often hit with chilling thoughts, flashbacks and memories of the event that caused the trauma to be etched to them.

- Developmental trauma disorder:

This disorder refers to the one where the person, mainly a child of age below 4 have trouble getting attached to any adult who tries to be caregivers. This usually occurs after mental or physical abuse or when the child is ignored or abandoned. It affects the mind of a little kid and make them traumatic. Sad but true.

The person is hit with unpredictable emotions and they are bombarded with flashbacks that refresh in their minds the memories of that trauma. People fail to manage their emotions that come from every nook and corner, uninformed. This puts stress on the human mind and often causes strained relationships, questionable behavior, gloomy mood, lack of interest in life and at times paranoia. This is what trauma seems like and how it affects people. Let's talk about its symptoms to identify it abruptly hence, to treat is quickly by activating your vagus nerve. The signs and symptoms are:

The physical symptoms:

- Headache

- Nausea

The other symptoms:

- The constant guilt

- Shame or fear

VAGUS NERVE

- Flashbacks
- Clandestine emergence of different emotions
- Intense feeling of loneliness
- Anger
- Hopelessness
- Sadness and despair
- Shock
- Denial
- Feeling of alienation
- Self-blame
- Insomnia
- Nightmares
- Fatigue
- Getting startled easily
- Aches and pain
- Muscle tension

And a lot more. This is the reason many wellness-experts call trauma a bad reaction of events that abundantly affect the mental health of a person and let them part ways with peace. The dominant method which helped the trauma patients is the stimulation of the vagus nerve. A very famous doctor, Doctor Scaer mentions in his book named, 'The Body Bears the Burden' that the traumatic memories are stored in a certain part of the brain that regulate the body. Therefore, the traumatic stress often occurs when any trigger causes the memory to play before them. Now, let's see how the vagus nerve helps get rid of the traumatic stress and helps the person to overcome the trauma:

The vagus nerve deals with human emotions to a great extent and when the long-term trauma strikes a person, just like anxiety and depression, it alleviates the trauma too, in no time. According to some experts, it is that magic fix which is required to eradicate any mental issue because big or small, it causes unrest to birth in mind and affect the entire system. Also, the brain does not function well when the unrest has strengthened its root in it. But everything is possible if you believe. Similarly, the vagus nerve combat and defeats the trauma easily. All that is needed to be done is to stimulate it through many stimuluses. Such as:

• Cold water –splashing cold water on the face or have a cold shower.

• Take care of your gut (mentioned for gazillionth time, I know.)

• Laugh aloud and a lot, you need endorphins, a lot of them.

• Breathe, take deep, belly breaths; the most famous way to activate the vagus nerve.

VAGUS NERVE

- Dance more! Yes! Shake a little and release it all. Ever seen any animal shaking from head to toe in a certain pattern? That's because it keeps them happy and stress free. Best way to deal with trauma, isn't it?

- Exercise for maintaining the vagal tone.

- Do what make you happy for real. This is also keeps you away from having traumatic stress.

As mentioned many times, the X cranial nerve is responsible to deal with the 'rest-and-digest' reflex. When the vagus nerve is stimulated, it causes the brain to get in action and order the inflammation reflex to die down immediately since it is the power hub of the body. Now the 'rest and digest' or 'tend or befriend' gets activated when the body is at rest and is not working furiously as it does throughout the day. Also, according to a research conducted by the experts from Amsterdam and US, the vagus nerve activation inhibit the pro-inflammatory cytokines which result in the elimination of the arthritis inflammation or any type of inflammation and that is the process which ultimately lowers the chances of obesity and cancer pathogenesis since these are the problems that are closely knitted with the inflammation disease. Moreover, there is a disease called Crohn's disease which refers to the inflammation of the digestive tract and it is responsible to cause diarrhea, pain in abdomen, weight loss, fatigue and other problems. Also, it is responsible to cause some diseases like some cancers, rheumatoid arthritis, atherosclerosis, periodontitis, and hay fever. A study has shown that inflammation is one of the contributors of epilepsy which is yet again treated easily by the vagus nerve stimulation, even when the anti-seizure medicines fail to help. This was approved by the FDA, prior to 2005.

Chromic pancreatitis is a part of inflammation diseases and it is also connected with gut. The pancreas is situated right behind the stomach and it is responsible to produce special protein enzymes that help the food to be digested. Moreover, the pancreas also controls the level of sugar in blood by secreting certain hormones. Now, the chronic pancreatitis occurs when inflammation occurs in pancreas. There are two types of pancreatitis, one is acute which lasts for a few days and usually don't come back and the chronic pancreatitis occurs when the inflammation is failed to be eliminated and keeps returning. Also, atop that it lasts for months and years and keeps growing severe. The chronic pancreatitis causes the permanent damage to the pancreas. The stones of calcium and also the cysts might occur in it too. This would cause blockage to occur in the pancreas which would prevent the digestive enzymes and fluid to be transferred to the stomach. The stomach would then have trouble digesting food and regulating the level of sugar in blood and keeping diabetes at bay. Also, it usually occurs in people aging from 30 to 40.

What possibly might be the causes of chronic pancreatitis? Well, they are mentioned below:

- Autoimmune disease

- A narrow pancreatic duct

- A blockage of the pancreatic duct (it carries enzymes from pancreas to small intestine).

- Cystic fibrosis which is a hereditary problem which involves mucus to be generated in the lungs.

- Hypercalcemia

- Hypertriglyceridemia

Well, other than these some other factors that are responsible to cause chronic pancreatitis are excessive alcoholism, smoking addiction and living in the tropical regions of Asia and Africa because there are chances of malnutrition according to some sources.

Well, you need to identify it before dealing with it and that is possible only when you would know the symptoms of chronic pancreatitis. Let's go through these various symptoms it shows:

- Nausea and vomiting

- Fatty, loose stale

- Excessive thirst

- Diarrhea

- Fatigue

- Upper abdominal pain

- Unexplained weight loss

- Shortness of breath

- Pancreatic juice would be found in abdomen

There are also some diseases that emerge as the symptoms of chronic pancreatitis, those are:

- Intestinal blockage

- Jaundice

- Internal bleeding

The pain also occurs which makes it unbearable to even breath let alone eat or drink.

Now, the chronic pancreatitis are often diagnosed by the following:

- X-rays

- MRI scan

- CT scan

- Ultrasound

There is also one magical cure for the Chronic pancreatitis that is the vagus nerve stimulation. Now let's discuss the cure!

The sensory information is carried by the vagus nerve to the CNS (Central Nervous System). The vagus nerve is a pathway basically where the bi-directional flow of information occurs from the gut to the brain and then from the brain to the gut. Hence, when chronic pancreatitis occurs, it knows ultimately that it has to send signals to the brain regarding the occurrence of the chronic pancreatitis. The pain during this condition is unbearable and the patient has to have a painkiller. But to stop both the disease to strengthen its root and the pain, one of the best cures is the vagus nerve stimulation by:

- Deep, belly breathing.

- Non-invasive transcutaneous vagus nerve stimulation

Now, by using these processes the pain sensitivity was seen decreasing. And, also, the gut motility was improved by these two methods. This proved that the modulation of the vagal tone index is really helpful in dealing with certain diseases involving gut problems and inflammation. The vagus nerve is a crucial part of the immune system and when stimulated, it proves to be really helpful in multiple diseases.

The Vagus Nerve and Irritable Bowel Syndrome

Irritable bowel syndrome or IBS is a very troublesome disease. It involves altered bowel habits such as:

- Bloating

- Gas

- Diarrhea

- Chronic constipation

- Severe pain and discomfort in abdomen

This disease is not necessarily a serious one or the one known as "life threatening" but the symptoms keeps the person troubled and causes unrest to develop in their mind. The bi-direction interaction between the gut and the brain thus, creating a brain-gut axis which keeps the balance maintained in the gastrointestinal tract. The main cause is still not discovered of this disease but a few sources say that the Irritable Bowel Syndrome is usually caused by certain allergies, stress (either physical or mental) and at times, it is reported to be transferred from one of the parents. The changes in one's lifestyle, environment and other areas are responsible to contribute in the occurrence of IBS. But there is a cure to IBS that would help you get rid of it without much effort. Want to know that? What are you waiting for then? Let's dive in!

any damage in the vagus nerve and examine it to see if it's the vagus nerve dysfunction that is causing the IBS to occur in the human being since it is the pathway between the gut and the brain that deals with all the aspects of the gastrointestinal tract. But if they fail to find any damage, they seek to activate the vagus nerve to maintain the vagal tone index. And that does all the work for them. The vagus nerve communicates with the brain about the problems occurring and brain jumps into action to solve all the issues including bloating, gas, abdominal pain and other symptoms IBS brings. The stomach acid runs low during IBS and the vagus nerve makes sure that this doesn't happen by causing the cells to release histamine which creates the stomach acid that the body needs to break the food down. Now, when the vagus nerve is activated through various ways –where non-invasive transcutaneous vagus nerve stimulation and deep belly breathing along with some exercise is mostly preferred– it provides various other benefits such as:

1. Promotes relaxation

2. Balances heart rate

3. Eradicates anxiety

VAGUS NERVE

4. Alleviate depression

5. Controls blood pressure

And many other countless benefits occur when one keeps the health of their vagus nerve in check and make sure that it is stimulating normally and effectively eradicating all the troubles that come their way. Well, it doesn't end here, there is more to the vagus nerve that you need to unveil!

# CHAPTER 9

THE NERVOUS SYSTEM

Recalling the earlier descriptions, the nervous system is actually comprised of two separate systems. One is the central nervous system (CNS), controlling the brain and the spinal cord, it's called central because it is the overriding controller of all bodily functions. The other is the peripheral nervous system (PNS), which is made of the many nerves that lead from the spinal cord and radiate throughout our bodies, extending to every extremity. Combined, these systems influence every organ and muscle, and all voluntarily and involuntarily actions, including reflexes, reactions, and responses.

Recall also that the nerves or neurons that form the substance and networks of the nervous system in the brain, the spinal cord and throughout the body, number in the billions, and form trillions of connections and interactions. Impulses that travel through and remain within the nervous system are electrical in nature, but with chemical reactions forwarding signals from one nerve to another. These are called synaptic connections.

Nervous System Overload

Considering the awesome number of nerves and their connections and interactions, it should come as no surprise that this complex nervous system can suffer from disruptions. Apart from a range of disruptive and debilitating physical conditions, including degenerative diseases, vascular and structural disorders, and infections, the nervous system can be overloaded, unable to function at full capacity and effectiveness.

When the nervous system becomes overloaded from stress, depression, anxiety, or from any number of factors that push the nervous system past a certain point, functionality becomes reduced and the body enters a state of fatigue. In these cases of system overload, fatigue cannot be traced to muscular deficiencies nor to depletion of glucose and other energy stores, and it is not resolved by rest. Something else is at work, affecting electro-chemical connectivity and reactivity.

There are many symptoms of nervous system overload, including persistent headaches, sudden onset headaches, and headaches that changes or may feel different, tingling sensations, and feelings of muscular weakness that cannot be attributed to physical exertion. Other symptoms may be loss of sight or experiencing double vision, loss of memory and impaired thinking ability, and a lack of coordination. In extreme situations, a person may suffer what is commonly called a nervous breakdown, left in a state of near immobility and unable to think clearly or rationally.

Central nervous system fatigue can occur as the result of excessive physical exercise. The molecular composition of the neurotransmitting chemicals that connect nerves to each other changes, slowing or altering the synaptic connections between the nerves, and this may slow or even block the neural connections between muscles and organs, and the brain and spinal cord.

Overcoming nervous system fatigue:

Several commonly available substances have been proven under medical testing to have a positive effect on preventing or reversing nervous system fatigue: coffee, carbohydrates, and amphetamine.

The caffeine in coffee acts to suppress production of adenosine, a chemical neurotransmitter that can induce fatigue. Athletes are cautioned to ingest coffee in moderation for optimal effect and for safety.

Ingestion of a combination of a readily-available carbohydrate. e.g., sugar, and an electrolyte, appears to increase plasma levels of glucose, a primary energy source. However, there is no increase noted of glycogen within muscles.

Taking amphetamines is commonly used by performance athletes to prevent or reverse central nervous system fatigue. It is known to alter the production of the neurotransmitters dopamine and norepinephrine, which play a role in inducing nervous system fatigue.

Chronic fatigue syndrome is characterized by physical fatigue that

VAGUS NERVE

is not caused by peripheral muscle fatigue. As with nervous system fatigue, it is persistent, not caused by exercise and not alleviated by rest. Subject suffering from this condition were unable to compete exercise tests, despite no obvious physical reason for their limitations.

The main cause of chronic fatigue syndrome has been traced to the central nervous system, where certain defects are slowing or otherwise altering neural connections. In other words, the muscles and organs of the body are intact and potentially fully functional, and it is the connecting electrical wires that are at fault. Precise medical treatments are still being explored, while the fatigue-relieving self-applications, like caffeine from coffee, carbohydrates with electrolytes, and amphetamines, are found to help along with motivational counseling.

Daily stress from a multitude of responsibilities and interests can lead to nervous system overload without any physical causes. Contemporary lifestyles include long work and study hours, insufficient time off, or a sense of guilt when time off is taken, an all-encompassing range of video and online distractions, plus personal and family responsibilities. In response, sleep deprivation may occur, multitasking becomes the standard work-and-activity management tool, and stress builds until it overwhelms the nervous system.

Situations that have reached nervous system overload may evoke the proverbial cup runneth over. One result may be activation of the sympathetic nervous system's fight or flight response, with surges of energy that are quickly depleted resulting in chronic fatigue, shortness of temper and irritability, and even in less extreme situations, a reduction in effectiveness and the absence of the satisfaction of fulfillment.

More extreme trauma may create nervous system overload. Involvement in an accident or a physical injury, for example, or a strong emotional shock, such as unexpectedly being fired or the ending of a close personal relationship. In these cases, as with the other situations, the parasympathetic response may cause overreaction. Consider the behavioral eccentricities of some extreme cases, including violent behavior.

How to respond to emotional, non-physical causes of nervous system overload?

The practical applications of the Polyvagal Theory may be successfully applied to diminish and perhaps eradicate the effects of nervous system overload. These include Yoga, meditation and managed breathing exercises, and the other procedures such as neck massage and cold facial treatments. The objective is to achieve vagal tone and activate the relaxation response and calming effects of the ventral vagal parasympathetic nervous system.

Degrees Of Stress

Stress. A word frequently used to describe everything from a simple sense of urgency to the extreme disabling conditions associated with long-term, overwhelming stress. We tend to think of stress as a modern affliction, resulting from the overload of obligations, media inputs, personal interactions both personal and professional, and everything brought to us online, such as social media, email, text messaging, streaming video, customized music playlists, news alerts and stories, magazine articles, eBooks and audiobooks, sports programs we can carry with us, and more.

Actually, people have always experienced stress due to any variety of outside influences, as well as internal sources, stemming from imagined or real concerns, fears, and worries. But, yes, today's environment seems to be overflowing with more than we can handle, leading to an almost infinite number of stimuli and distractions, engagements and commitments.

Consider the increased levels of our exposure to programming content and advertising. From historical print-only to radio, then the emergence and dominance of television. It was first local, then networked, national broadcasts, followed by cable broadcasts with huge numbers of watchable channels covering every interest. Add to this, today's technology-enabled out-of-home media that presents us with product information and advertising at the point-of-sale in supermarkets, drug stores and mass merchandisers, and even at the service stations to entertain and inform us while we're pumping gas. Of course, outdoor ads like billboards have been around for over a century, but today, a walk through a shopping mall will expose us to dozens, or sometimes hundreds, of electronic billboards, some of which are sophisticated enough to use facial recognition software to personalize ads as we approach. All-in-all, it's a lot to absorb, manage and digest.

Apart from this vast multitude of inputs, consider the many distractions and stimuli that the pressures society imposes upon us, plus the pressures we impose upon ourselves. Work, education, sports, even vacations can incite stress. How am I doing compared to my peers? Will I qualify for whatever you are aiming for? Do my parents love me? Does my spouse love me? Most of us manage to find a good number of concerns to think about, dwell on and worry about, and if we don't manage these concerns, they can become forms of stress in our lives.

In reality, stress is an emotional condition that psychologists classify into three degrees of seriousness on both emotional and physical levels:

1. Acute stress:

The most common form of stress, is frequently the result of intense, recent psychological pressures. These can be in the recent past, such as a scary, near-miss auto collision or concern over a just-ended difficult meeting, a tough exam or an interview just completed, and the outcome of which is of concern. Or, acute stress may be triggered by anticipation of a future event, like a sports challenge, a pending confrontation with a boss or a spouse, a scheduled operation, or dental procedure. Because acute stress tends to be short-term, even if extreme, it does not tend to cause serious side-effects or injury.

Emotional reactions to acute stress commonly include tension, anger and irritability, anxiety, and depression. Physical reactions may include stomach upset, loss of appetite, diarrhea or constipation, acid indigestion or chronic acid reflux (GERD). Also included can be tension headaches and migraine headaches, muscular tension, elevated heartbeat or heart palpitations, shortness of breath and lightheadedness or dizziness.

Many of these are symptoms of a defensive sympathetic nervous system response and may be alleviated by toning the vagus nerve and inducing the relaxation and social engagement responses of the parasympathetic nervous system. Meditation, Yoga stretches and poses, and managed deep breathing exercises can alleviate the

VAGUS NERVE

feelings and symptoms of acute stress.

2.   Episodic acute stress:

While ordinary acute stress is short-term and relatively harmless, when the patterns of stress are not occasional, or are due to multiple causes, a more extreme form of stress, called episodic acute stress, occurs. Episodic acute stress is longer-term, involves a multitude of stress-inducing factors, and is harder to manage and bring under control. It is often the result of an overloaded, excessively ambitious lifestyle, for example, the "Type A" personality defined by cardiologists (Friedman, M., and Rosenman. R., 1976). These are people who are excessively driven by often unrealistic goals, time urgency, and high levels of expected accomplishments. They tend to be aggressively ambitious, irritable, and impatient. Many are driven by a deep-seated insecurity and are outwardly overambitious in compensation to their insecurity.

Another type of person who suffers from episodic acute stress is the persistently worrying personality, like persons who have a pessimistic outlook on life, expect the worst, anticipate nothing working out. They are the antithesis of optimists. Unlike others who experience stress, these worry warts tend to be less angry and irritable, but are more likely to experience continuing bouts of depression or anxiety.

Emotional and physical symptoms of episodic acute stress are similar to those of acute stress, but being longer-term in nature, can induce more persistent and severe headaches, anxiety, depression, chest pain, and in the case of the Type A personalities, a greater propensity to develop heart disease.

Treatment of episodic acute stress is more difficult on several levels as the conditions it causes are more severe and chronic. Also, the personalities of these types of people make them resistant to behavioral and attitudinal changes. Type A personalities are convinced that their driven behavior is the right and only way, and others are lazy slackers. They believe nothing will get done without their excessive presence, pressure and micromanagement. Those who worry excessively are convinced that their concerns are realistic and necessary, believing that there is nothing positive to anticipate. In consequence, treatment to modify these attitudinal and behavioral extremes is complex, and often needs to be at the professional level.

3.   Chronic stress:

This is the long-term, potentially damaging stress of hopelessness. People experiencing this form of stress experience lives of continuing frustration, and see no way out and no ending to the trouble. Examples include women in loveless marriages and married men who realize they love someone else, who in turn, is also married and unavailable to them. It includes people in dead-end jobs they despise and who believe their lack of education, or their ethnicity, or their handicap or other physical characteristics will keep them from advancing or going elsewhere, and somewhere better. It can embrace people living in areas of violent conflict, whether in the shifting political turmoil in the Middle East, the poverty of certain African countries, or the gang-incited violence of some Central American countries or American inner cities. The common characteristics of chronic stress are senses of entrapment, a bleak future, and no way out.

The consequences of chronic stress can be severe, including

deep depression, a permanent state of anxiety, and unending hopelessness. Given its continuing nature, people with chronic stress may be unaware of its existence and its hold over them. They surrender to it, accepting it as normal, the way life is and was meant to be. Over time, chronic stress can leave the individual vulnerable to a range of diseases like mental illness, constant fatigue and muscular weakness, heart disease and a propensity to be suicidal. Chronic stress sufferers may be irritable, resentful of others who are not experiencing the same misery, and they may be subject to violent outbursts. Cases of someone going postal usually involve a person whose work situation was depressing, hopeless, and frustrating. These conditions can lead to reduced effectiveness on the job, thus accelerating a downward spiral, and leading to reprimands or termination. These actions, in turn, can become pivotal moments that trigger violent actions, often directed toward fellow workers.

Professional help is generally required to effectively pull a chronic stress sufferer back to a sense of normalcy, especially when they consider their unhappy condition to be inevitable. Treatment tends to require long term psychological counseling and therapy. The symptoms may have begun early in life and are deep seated. In addition, medical treatment may be required when the chronic stress has provoked long-term weakness, and muscular atrophy, and the onset of cardiovascular disease.

Panic And Hyperactivity

People who are subject to hyperactive behavior are most often diagnosed as having Attention Deficit Hyperactivity Disorder (ADHD). There is a tendency to experience bouts of panic, both short-term and longer-term, which affects 50% of adults and 35% of children who have been diagnosed with ADHD. The panic induces anxiety, and even at low levels it can exacerbate the customary ADHD behavioral effects: hyperactivity, nervousness, fidgeting and inability to sit still, as well as challenges to concentration and the completion of projects. In effect, hyperactivity and panic-induced anxiety tend to coexist. For example, an inability to focus or concentrate for a sustained period is characteristic of panic-induced anxiety and hyperactivity.

But there are symptoms that define panic-induced anxiety that exceed the normal bounds of ADHD. These include long term or chronic feelings of nervousness, a tendency to continuously worried, irritability, insomnia or other sleep disorders, frequent headaches and backaches not caused by physical strains, and fears of the unexpected and unknown.

Treatment to reduce or relieve panic-induced anxiety may be sought by discussing the symptoms with medical professionals. Counseling may advise self-evaluation to identify the triggers that create the panic, leading to recommended behavior modification. For example, if the making of deadlines is a source of panic reactions, the person may be encouraged to plan more carefully to allow more time to accomplish responsibilities.

Many of the symptoms of panic and anxiety may be due to activation of the sympathetic nervous system response, the call-to-action mechanism with its characteristic elevated heart and respiratory levels, and shutting down of digestion.

Separately, it is possible that medications prescribed for ADHD can cause panic or anxiety tendencies. Physicians can evaluate the

VAGUS NERVE

potential side effects of medications, and advise changing to those less likely to cause panic reactions.

CHAPTER 10

Causes Of Anxiety, Depression, And Inflammation

Relationship between inflammation, depression and anxiety

There is developing proof that inflammation can intensify or even offer ascent to burdensome side effects. The inflammatory response is a key part of our insusceptible framework. At the point when our bodies are attacked by microscopic organisms, infections, poisons, or parasites, the insusceptible framework initiates cells, proteins, and tissues, including the cerebrum, to assault these intruders. The principle technique is to stamp the harmed body parts, so we can give more consideration to them. Nearby inflammation makes the harmed parts red, swollen, and hot. At the point when the damage isn't confined, at that point, the framework ends up aggravated. These ace inflammatory variables offer ascent to "affliction practices." These incorporate physical, psychological and social changes. Normally, they wiped out individual encounters languor, weakness, slow response time, psychological impedances, and loss of craving. This star grouping of changes that happen when we are wiped out is versatile. It constrains us to get more rest to mend and stay disconnected so as not to spread diseases.

Be that as it may, a drawn-out inflammatory response can unleash ruin in our bodies and can put us in danger of depression and different sicknesses. There is a lot of proof cementing the connection between inflammation and depression. For instance, markers of inflammation are raised in individuals who experience the ill effects of depression contrasted with non-discouraged ones. Additionally, markers of inflammation can anticipate the seriousness of burdensome manifestations. An investigation that analyzed twins who offer 100 percent of similar qualities found that the twin who had a higher CRP fixation (a proportion of inflammation) was bound to create depression five years after the fact.

Specialists saw that their malignancy and Hepatitis C patients treated with IFN-alpha therapy (increments inflammatory response) likewise experienced depression. This treatment expanded the arrival of genius inflammatory cytokines, which offered ascend to lost hunger, rest aggravation, anhedonia (loss of joy), subjective impedance, and self-destructive ideation. The pervasiveness of depression in these patients was high. These outcomes add assurance to the inflammation story of depression.

Ensuing cautious investigations demonstrated that the expansion in the commonness of depression in patients treated with IFN-alpha was not just in light of the fact that they were wiped out. Utilizing a basic technique for infusing sound subjects with invulnerable framework intruders, specialists discovered higher paces of burdensome side effects during the ones which were presented contrasted with the fake treatment gathering. The subjects who were initiated to have an inflammatory response whined of indications, for example, negative state of mind, anhedonia, rest unsettling influences, social withdrawal, and intellectual weaknesses.

The connection between inflammation and depression is much increasingly strong for patients who don't react to flow antidepressants. Studies have demonstrated that treatment-safe patients will, in general, have raised inflammatory components circling at gauge than the responsive ones. This is clinically significant; a clinician can use a measure like CRP levels, which are a piece of a routine physical, to foresee the restorative response to antidepressants. In one examination, they found that expanded degrees of an inflammation particle preceding treatment anticipated poor response to antidepressants.

There are ecological components that reason inflammation and in this way, lift hazard for depression: stress, low financial status, or an agitated youth. Additionally, a raised inflammatory response prompts expanded affectability to stretch. The impact has been accounted for in numerous investigations in mice. For instance, mice that have gone under ceaseless flighty pressure have more elevated levels of inflammation markers. Strikingly, there are singular contrasts that make a few mice progressively impervious to push, in this way starting a more quiet safe response.

Depression is a heterogeneous disorder. Every patient's battle is extraordinary given their youth, hereditary qualities, and the affectability of their resistant framework, other existing real diseases, and their flow status in the public eye. Being on the disadvantageous finish of these measurements bothers our safe framework and causes incessant inflammation. The cerebrum is extremely responsive to these flowing inflammatory markers and starts "infection conduct." When the inflammation is drawn out by stressors or different vulnerabilities, the affliction conduct moves toward becoming depression.

Reasons for anxiety

Anxiety might be brought about by a state of mind, a physical condition, the effects of medications, or a blend of these. The specialist's underlying assignment is to check whether your anxiety is a manifestation of another ailment.

Current research on Anxiety Disorder

Much research is being done into what causes anxiety disorders. Specialists trust it includes a mix of components, including qualities, diet, and stress.

Investigations of twins recommend that hereditary qualities may assume a job. For instance, an investigation announced in plos ONE Trusted Source recommends the RBFOX1 quality might be engaged with the improvement of anxiety-related conditions, for example, summed up anxiety disorder. The creators accept that both hereditary and nongenetic variables have an influence.

Certain pieces of the cerebrum, for example, the amygdala and hippocampus, are additionally being considered. Your amygdala is a little structure somewhere inside your cerebrum that procedures risk. It cautions the remainder of your mind when there are indications of risk. It can trigger a dread and anxiety response. It appears to have an influence in anxiety disorders that include dread of explicit things, for example, felines, honey bees, or suffocating.

Your hippocampus may likewise influence your danger of building up an anxiety disorder. It's a locale of your cerebrum that is associated with putting away recollections of undermining occasions. It seems, by all accounts, to be littler in individuals who've encountered kid misuse or served in battle.

What causes anxiety disorders?

Anxiety is a psychological wellness condition that can cause sentiments of stress, dread, or pressure. For certain individuals, anxiety can likewise cause fits of anxiety and extraordinary physical side effects, similar to chest torment.

The definite reasons for anxiety disorders are obscure. As indicated by the National Institute of Mental Health, specialists accept that a mix of hereditary and ecological variables may assume a job. Cerebrum science is likewise being concentrated as a conceivable reason. The zones of your mind that control your dread response might be included.

Anxiety disorders frequently happen close by other psychological wellness conditions, for example, substance misuse and depression. Numerous individuals attempt to facilitate the side effects of anxiety by utilizing liquor or different medications. The help these substances give is brief. Liquor, nicotine, caffeine, and different medications can exacerbate an anxiety disorder.

Anxiety disorders are unimaginably normal. They influence an expected 40 million individuals in the United States, as indicated by the Anxiety and Depression Association of America.

What causes anxiety and anxiety disorders can be muddled. Almost certainly, a blend of components, including hereditary qualities and ecological reasons, assume a job. In any case, plainly a few occasions, feelings, or encounters may make side effects of anxiety start or may aggravate them. These components are called triggers.

Anxiety triggers can be distinctive for every individual, except numerous triggers, are normal among individuals with these conditions. A great many people discover they have numerous triggers. Be that as it may, for certain individuals, anxiety assaults can be activated for reasons unknown by any stretch of the imagination.

Therefore, it's imperative to find any anxiety triggers that you may have. Distinguishing your triggers is a significant advance in overseeing them. Continue perusing to find out about these anxiety triggers and what you can do to deal with your anxiety.

What are the anxiety triggers

Health Issues

A wellbeing analysis that is annoying or troublesome, for example, malignancy or a constant sickness, may trigger anxiety or exacerbate it. This kind of trigger is ground-breaking on account of the prompt and individual sentiments it produces.

You can help lessen anxiety brought about by medical problems by being proactive and drawn in with your primary care physician. Conversing with a specialist may likewise be valuable, as they can enable you to figure out how to deal with your feelings around your analysis.

Medications

Certain remedy and over-the-counter (OTC) medications may trigger indications of anxiety. That is on the grounds that dynamic fixings in these medications may make you feel uneasy or unwell. Those emotions can set off a progression of occasions in your brain and body that may prompt extra side effects of anxiety.

Prescriptions that may trigger anxiety include:

•Birth control pills

•Cough and blockage medications

•Weight misfortune medications

Converse with your PCP about how these medications make you feel and search for an elective that doesn't trigger your anxiety or decline your side effects.

Caffeine

Numerous individuals depend on their morning cup of joe to wake up; however, it may really trigger or exacerbate anxiety. As per one investigation in 2010Trusted Source, individuals with frenzy disorder and social anxiety disorder are particularly touchy to the anxiety-inciting effects of caffeine.

VAGUS NERVE

Work to curtail your caffeine admission by substituting noncaffeinated alternatives at whatever point conceivable.

Skipping Suppers

When you don't eat, your glucose may drop. That can prompt anxious hands and a thundering stomach. It can likewise trigger anxiety.

Eating adjusted suppers is significant for some reasons. It furnishes you with vitality and significant supplements. In the event that you can't set aside a few minutes for three suppers per day, solid tidbits are an extraordinary method to anticipate low glucose, sentiments of nervousness or fomentation, and anxiety. Keep in mind, nourishment can influence your disposition.

Negative Reasoning

Your mind controls quite a bit of your body, and that is positively valid with anxiety. When you're vexed or baffled, the words you state to yourself can trigger more prominent sentiments of anxiety.

On the off chance that you will, in general, utilize a lot of negative words when considering yourself, figuring out how to refocus your language and sentiments when you start down this way is useful. Working with an advisor can be fantastically useful with this procedure.

Budgetary Concerns

Stresses over setting aside cash or having an obligation can trigger anxiety. Sudden bills or cash fears are triggers, as well.

Figuring out how to deal with these sorts of triggers may need looking for expert support, for example, from a monetary guide. Feeling you have a buddy and a guide in the process may facilitate your worry.

Gatherings Or Get-Togethers

In the event that a room brimming with outsiders doesn't seem like fun, you're not the only one. Occasions that expect you to make casual chitchat or associate with individuals you don't know can trigger sentiments of anxiety, which might be analyzed as a social anxiety disorder.

To help facilitate your stresses or unease, you can continually bring along a friend when conceivable. But at the same time, it's critical to work with an expert to discover methods for dealing with stress that make these occasions increasingly sensible in the long haul.

Struggle

Relationship issues, contentions, differences — these contentions would all be able to trigger or compound anxiety. On the off chance that contention especially triggers you, you may need to learn compromise systems. Additionally, converse with an advisor or other emotional well-being master to figure out how to deal with the sentiments these contentions cause.

Stress

Day by day stressors like congested driving conditions or missing your train can cause anybody anxiety. Yet, long haul or constant pressure can prompt long haul anxiety and compounding manifestations, just as other medical issues.

Stress can likewise prompt practices like skipping dinners, drinking liquor, or not getting enough rest. These elements can trigger or intensify anxiety, as well.

Treating and avoiding pressure regularly requires getting the hang of methods for dealing with stress. A specialist or advocate can enable you to figure out how to perceive your wellsprings of stress and handle them when they become overpowering or hazardous.

Open Occasions Or Exhibitions

Open talking, talking before your chief, performing in a challenge, or even simply perusing so anyone might hear is a typical trigger of anxiety. In the event that your activity or diversions require this, your primary care physician or advisor can work with you to learn approaches to be increasingly agreeable in these settings.

Additionally, uplifting comments from companions and associates can enable you to feel increasingly good and sure.

Individual Triggers

These triggers might be hard to distinguish, yet a psychological well-being authority is prepared to enable you to recognize them. These may start with a smell, a spot, or even a tune. Individual triggers remind you, either intentionally or unknowingly, of an awful memory or awful accident in your life. People with post-awful pressure disorder (PTSD) as often as possible experience anxiety triggers from ecological triggers.

Distinguishing individual triggers may require some serious energy,

Dr. Jason Rosenberg

yet it's significant so you can figure out how to conquer them.

VAGUS NERVE

CHAPTER 11

WHAT HAPPENS IF THE VAGUS NERVE IS DAMAGED?

As we have observed, it is possible that the vagus nerve can be damaged. The nerve can be damaged due to excessive pressure on the nerve or due to stress. Continuous stimulation of the nerve can lead to damage if it is not done in the right way. There are also surgical medical procedures that can lead to the nerve being cut or damaged by surgical instruments. In either case, nerve damage can cause serious problems for the patient.

If your nerve is completely damaged, you may experience some of the following problems.

- Speaking or Voice Problems: Damaged nerves can affect the voice box, which may lead to a wheezy voice or difficulty in speaking.

- Trouble Eating and Drinking: Any damage to the vagus

nerve may affect how your throat muscles operate. Given that they are responsible for swallowing food, you will eventually experience problems when taking food or swallowing water. In essence, vagus nerve damage mainly affects the gag reflex. As we have already observed, the gag reflex is responsible for ensuring that the food pipe is opened up to allow the swallowing of foods as you eat.

- Loss of Hearing or Pain in the Ear: There are high chances that your hearing will be affected in case your vagus nerve gets damaged. Any damage to the vagus nerve may lead to pain in the ear, given that the nerve extends to the outermost part of the ear. The nerve is also linked directly to your eardrums. This shows that any damage to the nerve may affect your hearing ability and may lead to loss of hearing or may cause pain in the ears.

- Affected Heart Rate and Blood Pressure: When your vagus nerve is affected, you must expect significant changes in your heart rate and blood pressure. The vagus nerve is the extension of the autonomic nervous system that directly links the heart to the brain. This means that any action that may affect the vagus can directly impact on the coordination between the heart and the brain. This may cause major damage to your heart and definitely affect the heart rate. When the heart rate is affected, then the blood pressure is also affected. The blood pressure is maintained by a steady heartbeat. If the heartbeat jumps up a bit, the blood pressure also fluctuates.

- Abdominal Pains and Stomach Pains: Damage to the vagus nerve often leads to decreased stomach acids. This means that you may experience some problems with food digestion. There is a level of stomach acids that should be maintained at all times. Any damage to the vagus nerve means that the glands responsible for the production of stomach acids do not get signals that start the process of acid production. Further, any damage to the vagus nerve may also affect abdominal muscles. It is the vagus nerve in conjunction with the nervous system that stimulates the abdominal areas. The nerve is responsible for sexual arousal because it extends to all the sexual parts. The nerve sends signals that start ovulation and other sexual activities. If the nerve is damaged, the chances are that a person may experience some abdominal pains. This is particularly true in ladies.

Communication Effects of Vagus Nerve Damage

The auricular vagus nerve is the nerve that links the central vagus nerve from the brain with the ear. The auricular vagus never ends on the back skin of the wear, extending a variety of smaller nerves on the ear. One of the important roles played by this nerve is sensory action. In simple terms, the nerve is responsible for collecting communication senses and sending signals to the brain for interpretation. If the nerve was not in place, it would be a big problem for most people to perceive communication. Some of the problems that would occur in your communication if the vagus nerve was damaged include:

Inability to Perceive Words: We perceive words during communication, not only from our hearing but also from observation. When you look at a person, you can tell what they are saying by looking at their lips. In many ways, these observations help us link what a person is saying to their voice, making communication easy and flawless. However, in a case where the vagus nerve is completely damaged, the sensory aspect of our

VAGUS NERVE

hearing is lost. We are unable to place a direct relationship to the voice and movements of the mouth from the other person. This brings a lot of complications in the communication process. It is important to have a clear sense when speaking to a person so that you can perceive what they are saying even when you cannot hear the words directly.

Inability to Perceive the Direction of Voices: One way that human beings maintain a clear focus in life is through the ability to sense the direction of the voice. While you may hear voices, without knowing the direction and distinctly separating one sound from another, you may be in huge trouble. The balanced sense of voices helps a person maintain stability while standing or walking. Any imbalances in the hearing aspects may cause a person to lean towards one side. If the vagus nerves in one year are damaged, this may force a person to tilt to one side, where the vagus sense is active.

Being in a position to sense the direction of a voice contributes to a large extent in the communication process. For instance, in a room where you have to communicate with several people at a go, you may not be able to function appropriately if your ears fail to sense the direction from which the sound is coming. If you work at a pace where communication flows through a chain, you may have problems when trying to link up the chain.

The most dangerous scenario in vagus nerve failure would come when you are crossing streets. Knowing the direction of sound is important in helping a person perceive warnings from cars while walking on the streets. If you do not know where a sound is coming from, you may easily be involved in road accidents. You may take longer to recognize cars coming your way, or you may easily confuse the direction of a warning sound and run directly into the same danger.

All these factors show the importance of the vagus nerve in facilitating communication. It is important to ensure that the nerve remains healthy so that it does not affect communication in any way. Failure of the nerve may lead to many problems at a personal level.

Inability to Perceive High Volumes: Another danger that a person suffering from a damaged vagus nerve faces is the inability to perceive volumes. Although the person might be able to hear, they lose the sense of detecting the volume range. This means that the patient may be exposed to very high volumes without noticing. This is a big danger given that the high volumes may lead to eardrum damage. The sensory aspect of the vagus nerve is very vital in protecting the ear from noise and high volumes. If your sensory nerves are completely damaged, you fail to differentiate sounds and volumes. The ear does not send the necessary signals to the brain. This leaves the patient exposed to dangerous situations that may lead to the damage of the eardrums and eventually cause a total loss of hearing.

If you are unable to perceive volumes, you also miss a lot in communication. When communicating with a person, you need to perceive their actions and pay attention to tonation. If a person raises their voice during an argument or a debate, you can perceive from the raised tone that the person is getting emotional. Such clues can only be detected if your nerves play the role of detecting communication flaws. If your vagus nerve is entirely damaged, you are not in a position to understand communications that result from voice variations. This is another reason why you must protect your vagus nerve from any damage.

Pain in the Ear: Another effect of the damaged vagus nerve in communication is constant pain in the ear. This does not affect your hearing as much, but continuous pain may lead to further complications. If you constantly feel pain in the ear or in the veins that extend to the ear, the chances are that your vagus nerve has been damaged. People who suffer from damaged auricular nerve usually feel pain from the ear, extending all the way to the neck. The auricular nerve links up from the lower part of your neck, this means that any damage to your ear nerves may affect your neck and your head. Damages to the vagus nerve in the ear section may lead to pain in the neck and headaches constantly. These factors affect your concentration. This type of pain may lead to hearing problems in the long run too. The patient is likely to feel as if the ears are clouded with dust. It is often difficult for the patient to perceive communications due to the pain and discomfort. Most people who suffer from damaged nerves stay in a state of discomfort and unease for a long time. When they speak, they have to strain thinking that other people may also not perceive the communication effectively.

The Response of the Body When the Nerve Damage

The vagus nerve serves a large part of our internal and external bodies. There are key body parts that will lose their sense if the vagus nerve is damaged. We have already established that the vagus nerve provides two components of sensory response. The somatic component mainly refers to the external sensory sensation provided by the nerve. The external senses of the vagus nerve are mainly felt on the skin or in the muscles. In areas of the body where the vagus nerve extends to the skin, you are able to feel a sensation associated with the nerve. A good example is an ear, where the auricular nerves extend to the surface of the ears.

The other component of sensory provided by the vagus nerve is known as the visceral sense. This mainly refers to sensations felt in the internal body organs. In essence, the vagus nerve has control over very key internal body organs and is responsible for the response of such organs during moments when the body is required to take action.

A damaged vagus nerve may affect both somatic and visceral components of the body. The sensory components provide by this nerve are not only important in keeping a person alert, but they also facilitate internal body processes. This means that the nerve plays a central role in detecting changes in the body and also enhances the production of necessary hormones. If these sensory properties of the nerve are cut off due to vagus nerve damage, it would be impossible for any person to lead a normal life. As we have observed, some of the problems associated with vagus nerve damage are due to sensory failure. For instance, in a case where a person has undergone vagotomy, the chances are that the vagus nerve may fail to stimulate intestinal glands to secret stomach acids when they are needed. As a result, a person may suffer acid reflux, vomiting, nausea, among other conditions. We have also seen that individuals who suffer from damaged vagus nerve may constantly lack appetite or vomit all the food soon after eating. All these factors are related to the fact that the glands required to secrete enzymes and acids do not get the right signal from the nervous system. Any

VAGUS NERVE

damage to the vagus nerve may affect the following body parts and organs.

The Ear: The sense of hearing may largely be damage. This is because the auricular vagus nerve extends to the outer skin of the ear. This means that, if a person has a damaged neve, the ears may not be able to feel any sense of touch or sometimes perceive sounds. The vagus nerve to the ear extends to the ear canal. This means that the ear canal may be damaged even without a person sensing the pain. All these factors affect a person's communication, as we have seen above. If you want to maintain your hearing, you must protect your vagus nerve from damage. We have already looked at some of the causes of ear canal damage. In your efforts to try and protect your ear from getting damaged, you can use the points mentioned. We will also look at some natural ways of protecting your vagus nerve as we proceed.

Throat: The other body part that may be affected by vagus nerve damage is the throat. The vagus nerve to the ear extends to the throat. It is the vagus nerve that supports gag flex, which is an important physiological process in the body. Without gag flex, it is impossible for any person to eat and swallow food. The damage to your vagus nerve my affect throat muscles leading to failure in the mouth and actions in the mouth.

Visceral Sensation for the Larynx: The larynx (voice box) is an important organ that plays a central role in your communication. The response of this body part primarily depends on the well-being of the vagus nerve. Even if you try speaking, you may not succeed as long as your vagus nerve is completely damaged. In other words, a damaged vagus nerve may directly affect your speech. Some people who have damaged vagus nerves produce wheezy voices while others completely fail to speak. The extent to which the nerve is damaged determines the level of communication. If the damage is severe, a person may be completely inaudible when they speak.

Sensory Effect for the Esophagus: The esophageal is the extension of the vagus nerve to the esophagus. This nerve is very important in sending communications to the brain and back to the esophagus. The vagus nerve plays an important role in directing food down to the stomach. If the esophagus does not have a sensory effect, then the food swallowed may not move down to the stomach. The esophagus is always in constant constriction to help the movement of food as it is lowered into the stomach. All these movements are directly supported by the subconscious actions of the vagus nerve. If the vagus nerve is damaged, there would be a problem since a person would have to consciously strain to push the food into the stomach.

Sensory Action in the Lungs: The lungs are an integral part of your being and are part of the body that are affected by any damage to the vagus nerve. Lungs do not only help you breathe, but they also affect the flow of fresh air into the brain. The movement of fresh air into the lungs, to the brain and back out is influenced by the vagus nerve. It is the nerve that determines the rate of contraction and expansion of the blood vessels. Although such actions happen subconsciously, any damage to the vagus nerve may directly affect your breathing, leading to far-reaching effects in your normal life.

Sensory Action in the Trachea: Also known as the windpipe, the trachea is an important body organ that connects your throat to your lungs. We have mentioned that the gag reflex in your throat is responsible for the separation of food and air at the throat. You have probably have been in a position where tiny pieces of food found their way into the trachea. Even if it is a very tiny piece of food, it leads to extensive coughing and suffocation. If action is not taken in a few minutes, a person may be chocked to death. This explains how delicate the trachea can be. The vagus nerve sensory action helps to distinguish the esophagus from the trachea. Through the sensory action of the vagus nerve, foods are directly moved to the esophagus while air is directed to the trachea. The sensory action of the vagus nerve helps manipulate the trachea to help control to counter movement of fresh air in and used air out. All these aspects would be affected in case the vagus nerve is damaged. The trachea would fail to coordinated the activities that lead to easy breathing, hence creating complications.

Sensory Action to the Heart: The heart is probably the most important organ of the human body. The fact that its actions are directly coordinated by the vagus nerve sends chills on the thought of a damaged vagus nerve. The pulmonary and cardiac extensions of the vagus nerve directly coordinate the activities of the heart. Like all the other parasympathetic actions of the vagus nerve, the activities of the heart are controlled subconsciously. In other words, the vagus nerve is able to coordinate the actions of the heart without your perceptions. The key sensory activities of the vagus nerve include the contraction of heart muscles, constriction of blood veins, and the communication between the heart and the brain. All these actions can directly impact the heart rate and blood pressure, as we have already observed. Any damage to the vagus nerve may mean disruption to the regular activities carried out by the heart. Some of the regular activities carried out may stop or may adopt an irregular pattern. We have seen that overstimulation of the vagus nerve may lead to a drop in blood pressure or an increase in heart rate. If this is the case, a damaged nerve may also lead to a serious drop in heart pressure. These actions are likely to cause fainting. The case gets worse if the vagus nerve is completely damaged. In this case, a person may get into a permanent state of unconsciousness.

VAGUS NERVE

Dr. Jason Rosenberg

CHAPTER 12

Activating the Vagus Nerve

Through breathing exercises, cold blasts, holding a healthy intestine, and some other basic activities, you can tone your vagal pathways. Modern medicine treats specific organs as part of the disease and overlooks the point that your brain plus central nervous system tells you how to proceed.

Your organs often send a status check with the vagus nerve to your brain to report exactly how it all works. It's a street in two ways. If all goes well, your brain will maintain the status quo. If an organ struggles, it can mean even more information for your brain. Your vagus nerve carries the signal to your organs from your brain to slow down until it's time for your body to spring to action.

Inflammation Tension and Fight or Flight Immune Response

Because the vagus nerves are involved in a lot of things, they must

VAGUS NERVE

work properly. Continue reading to learn how, through vagal toning, you can help your vagus nerve. There is a relationship between respiration and pulse rate, which is modulated by the nerve of the vagus. It is precisely for this reason that regular yoga practice reduces general stress.

Breathing yoga and then breathing guided exercises will calm your heart rate to minimize your blood pressure. Breathing exercises improved overall vagal tone and in an experimental group, properly handled prehypertension. Slower breathing exercises improved autonomic characteristics in healthy participants in a single study.

It wasn't fast breathing.

That's how quickly your body thinks you're running from predators.

That sets off the alarm bells of your body and causes a response to stress.

Breathing kit for S.O.S. Tries breathing box when you're panicking or about to blow a gasket.

Inhale a four-count.

Keep a count of four.

Exhale a count of four.

Hang on to a count of four.

Repeat until the controls have your hands available.

Trace your finger in the air in a square format the first few times.

It'll help you remember when you're frazzled how to get it done.

The gradual development of your respective lungs signals to slow down to your heart, through your whole nervous system. Your vagus nerve connects all these releases and signals acetylcholine, a calming substance that you can use relaxation methods to give yourself a go at any moment. The vagus response, which delays the activation of the sympathetic nervous system, becomes familiar with the chilly tones.

Constant cold blasts reduce indicators of pressure dramatically.

Chilly exposure helped alleviate anxiety and depression symptoms, possibly modulated by the nerve of the vagus. It stimulates digestion by revitalizing the vagal pathways. Due to anxiety, when the digestion of rats slowed down, cold stimulation reactivated the stomach nerves and got the products going again.

It all happened through vagal paths.

Keep your gut happy. Have you ever learned about the axis of the gut? This describes how your digestive system's microorganisms talking to your brain. Your microbiota is the ecosystem of your body and your skin's pleasant bacteria. They usually talk about the germs in your colon and intestines when someone talks about the microbiome.

Because the microbiome research is building up, the medical community is developing more and more approaches that impact the entire body. Investigating the relationship between the microbiome and the spirits is increasing, and interaction between the gut and the mind depends on the vagus nerve-surprise.

VAGUS NERVE

Human and animal models research to support the notion that a prosperous microbiome reduces tension and raises your mood. Rodents that supplemented with different probiotic strains reported reductions in anxiety and stress markers, but not in animals whose were cut vagus nerves before experimentation. Researchers see the beneficial effects of probiotics on people's moods.

Good females who have eaten fermented food for four weeks have shown positive changes in brain activity, particularly in the mental components that manage emotions and feelings. Through animal studies and probably from what scientists know about the vagus nerve, you can well believe that the gut-brain communication here occurs in the vagus nerve.

The very first stage to get through when you have an anxious stimulus is the person who addresses interpersonal interaction-oral language, body language, facial firmness, and several other non-verbal signals. When the stimulus is simply too powerful to reason, the fight or flight reaction triggers your brain. If this fails, the most primitive reaction of fear is probably to play the perception frozen.

If you realize that your fear is irrational, you can use protective measures to stop the panic at the very first level and prevent your brain from reacting with fighting or flight.

Let me share a few things that you can do.

Choose relaxing voices.

One of the ways children experience this phenomenon hardwired.

Children are measurably calmed by the prosodic (singing song), which is also known as mothers.

Changing your speech tone also works for adults.

Guided meditations are accompanied by a slow, rhythmic overall tone, whether personally or even registered.

Using the voice as a source of calming coaxes the mind more easily into a relaxed state than a normal chat.

Train your safety indicators You can train your mind to feel safe with some practice.

Protection measures protect your fear and anxiety from kick-in reactions.

One way to do this is to make your place safe or happy while you are calm.

To do this, you imagine you're in a place where you're completely comfortable, contented, and peaceful.

Use as much sensory information as possible? View sights, sounds, smells, and so on.

Practice this specific visualization often.

In this way, if you begin to feel angry or frightened, you can start a safe place without much effort.

If you want it, it's there.

Check for your myelin.

VAGUS NERVE

The vagus nerve is myelinated, which could mean it is filled with an extra fat protective layer that isolates it and enables the signals to move efficiently.

If myelin breaks down on any nerve, the nerve does not do the job.

Surgically implanted vagus stimulator

The vaguely implanted nerve triggers the immune system of the body when you fight.

Physicians use this knowledge to treat inflammatory problems, revitalizing the vagus with pharmaceuticals and electricity.

Surgically, physicians place electric vagus nerve stimulators in individuals with severe depression and epilepsy because they dampen the effect of inflammation.

You should tone the vagus nerve of your baby.

Several factors play into the vagal tone of the child. Babies born early, or mothers born during pregnancy who have anxiety and depression, are of low vagal tone.

Don't worry if you go through a few things during pregnancy. You can help to tone the vague ways of your baby with regular connections and loving attention.

Strong showers almost certainly should wait until the junior is old enough to agree.

Infant massage and kangaroo treatment (holding skin-to-skin baby) develop the vagal tone of the babies during infant years.

Dr. Jason Rosenberg

If your children go beyond childhood, you can use these methods for toning the vagus, such as cold blows and breathing techniques in the bath.

A massage and a few minutes of goosebumps in your bathroom probably deserve to be considered, because the benefits of vagal nerve toning also extend to every major organ in your body and have come back.

VAGUS NERVE

Dr. Jason Rosenberg

CHAPTER 13

Alternative Ways To Activate Vagus Nerve

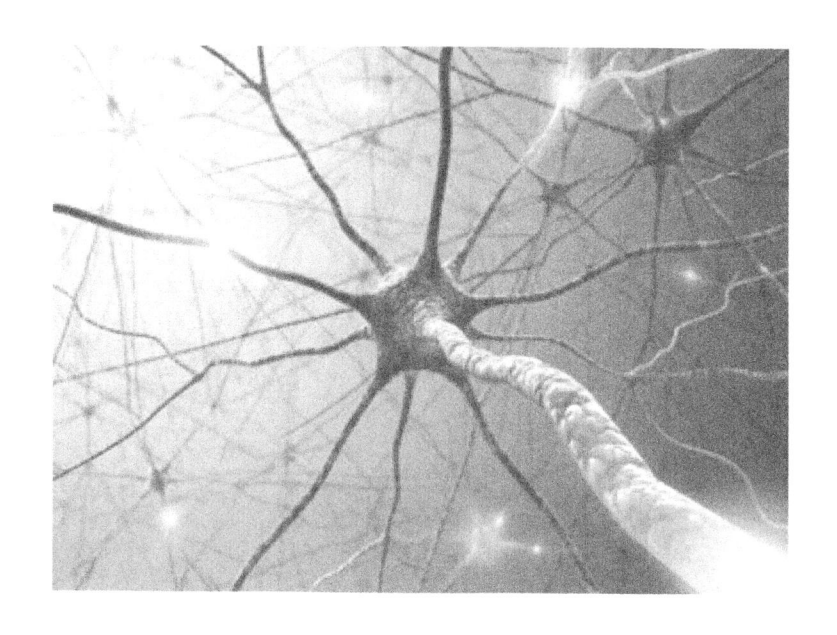

Human Energy Layers

In Divine Love spiritual healing, it does not matter how an illness is contracted or where it is located in the physical body. Removing the harmful energy that causes illness is important, however. That energy can exist in multiple layers and at various locations in the body. The harmful energy is intertwined with the energies of the soul, the mind, and the physical body.

Harmful energy attracts additional harmful energy. When the harmful energy builds up to a high enough level, it is difficult to remove through healing modalities that do not use Divine Love.

Everyone's body has hundreds of energy layers, both inside and outside the body. The first layer in a healthy person is located outside the body about 4 inches from the skin surface. Ordinarily, the body heals energetically from the outside to the inside of a person's core being. Each energy layer is capable of interacting with thoughts and actions.

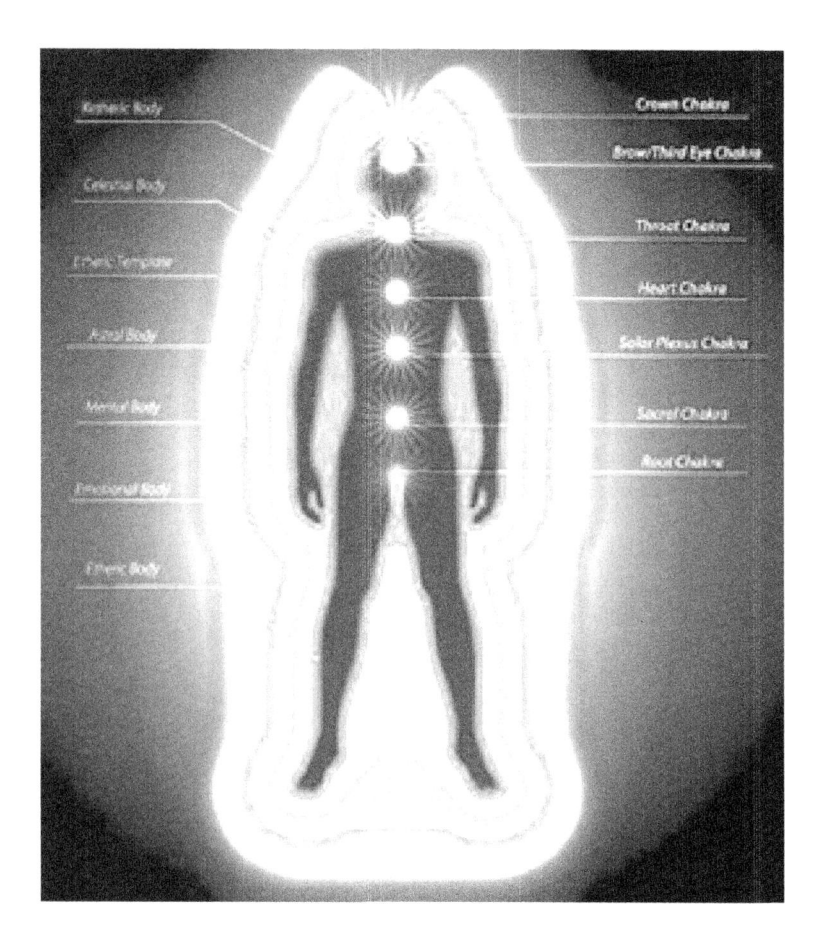

The layers expand and contract as a function of breathing and wellness. When a person breathes in, he compresses his layers toward his core; when he breathes out, his layers expand to their normal position. A person experiencing mental or emotional trauma may project energy layers several feet from the body. Or, energy layers may collapse on one side of the body, frequently causing severe pain.

When energy layers are allowed to expand in an uncontrolled fashion, we begin to absorb emotional energy from other people that can adversely impact our own energy layers. Over time, when someone has severe emotional problems, the layers can become very dense "clumps" of emotional energy that can also prevent proper functioning.

The healing approach used for these two distinct problem sources is very important. We found that about half of all illness cases manifest from stored emotional energy. If these emotions are not released, over time they will literally "plug" your energy layers.

When energy layers become plugged, cells lose their ability to communicate with each other. The cells may die, they may begin to mutate, or they may interrupt body functions. This process eventually produces a variety of symptoms that can become life-threatening diseases.

People may or may not be aware of their energy blockages. Blockages caused by post-traumatic stress may be complex; other illnesses are more easily recognized when they originate from a purely physical cause. An underlying cause can be introduced at any time in a person's life, even genetically introduced at conception.

Dr. Jason Rosenberg
Activating the Vagus Nerve

Parasympathetic System

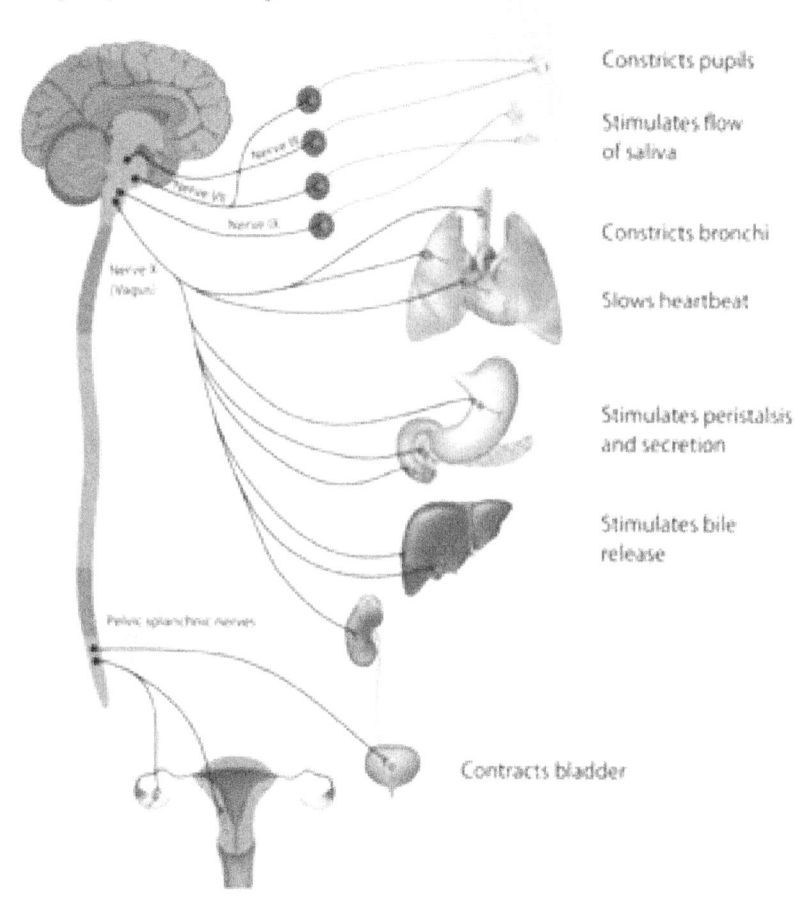

- Constricts pupils
- Stimulates flow of saliva
- Constricts bronchi
- Slows heartbeat
- Stimulates peristalsis and secretion
- Stimulates bile release
- Contracts bladder

Divine Love, the universal energy from the Creator, exists everywhere in a neutral state. When you initiate a petition, your spirit activates the energy of Divine Love and then your spirit utilizes Divine Love to effect a change in your body. Your spirit works with Divine Love unless you disconnect from Divine Love before your healing is complete. Should this occur, Divine Love returns to a neutral state and nothing more happens until you reconnect your system to Divine Love. Now you understand the importance of always staying connected.

Harmful energy can exist in some or all of your energy layers. When dealing with a systemic blood disease or sepsis, it is likely that all layers have been contaminated by the harmful energy causing the illness.

For those of you exhibiting major inflammation in your body, you should note that there is a spiritual basis for this. Your spirit and mind interact and cause energetic and physical friction, resulting in inflammation (and sometimes swelling) that does not go away. People with weight control problems will see improvements when they use petitions correctly to eliminate the inflammation in their bodies.

Occasionally, people report that their symptoms return after a few days. This usually occurs either because they stopped the petitions before healing was complete or they disconnected from Divine Love.

Staying Connected to Divine Love

Let us first understand what is meant by accelerated healing. There are three fairly obvious factors to consider:

- When you have multiple illnesses, it should be obvious that it will take longer for you to heal than if you had just one straightforward problem. If you are very ill, it may take your body significant time to process the energy of Divine Love in your body.

- A person comfortable with the spiritual healing process and who has a single symptom frequently experiences instantaneous healing. Others may take anywhere from hours to days to achieve the same level of healing, so please don't compare your progress to others. You are a unique individual and your Spirit knows exactly what needs to be done.

- If you are distracted or become unloving towards yourself or others, you may unknowingly disconnect yourself from Divine Love, and then all healing ceases. Healing does not resume until you re-initiate that Divine Love connection.

By always staying connected to Divine Love, you will transition your entire system into a spiritual mode where you will be living a life of Divine Love. What does it mean to live life this way? Very simply, even when chaos erupts around you, you will be able to function without being driven by your emotions. And, you will be able to function with clarity while others become upset and lose their objectivity.

Also, each time you audibly state your intent to reconnect to Divine Love, you enable Divine Love to bypass any resistance to change that may come from your subconscious mind. This is vitally important to facilitate healing.

Remember that if you perceive that a physical symptom has left or is diminished, but it suddenly returns, it is quite likely that you have disconnected from Divine Love.

VAGUS NERVE

Feeling Divine Love Energy

If you are experiencing energy healing for the first time, you may not know the many ways Divine Love energy feels in your body. You might feel heat, a tingle, a vibration, a cooling effect, or even see swirling energy around your body; it is all normal.

Since everyone has angelic support, some people find it more assuring to ask their angels to assist them in processing Divine Love. Years ago, we always invited the Angels to participate. Now, with the energy of Divine Love so high, Angelic participation is optional. Choose to work whichever way brings you the most comfort.

The simple act of accepting Divine Love fills your body with the right amount of Divine Love energy to heal your system. There is always enough Divine Love for the most complex healing, so you no longer need group support. You are self-healing in conjunction with the Creator's Divine Love.

CHAPTER 14

EXERCISES FOR THE VAGUS NERVE

The same can happen if we exercise our Vagus nerve consistently. We can strengthen

The Vagus nerve is effective in fighting against autoimmune disorders such as rheumatoid arthritis, chronic inflammation, reduces blood pressure, regulates the heart rate which is crucial for cardiovascular health and improves gut health.

Good vagal tone tremendously improves psychological health and is good for stress management.

Increasing vagal tone can be realized by incorporating physical exercise and other types of exercises to build a consistent exercise routine and keep the Vagus nerve healthy.

Breathing

VAGUS NERVE

Breathing is essential to our survival and one of the ways that we can achieve better health and regulating our nervous system. Slow, concentrated breathing is an easy and good way to stimulate the Vagus nerve and strengthen the vagal tone. Your breathing for stimulation can reduce anxiety, stress, anger, and inflammation. This is activating your parasympathetic nervous system's relaxation response.

Slow abdominal breathing, also known as diaphragmatic breathing, can be done anywhere and anytime to stimulate the Vagus nerve immediately and diminish stress responses associated with the sympathetic nervous system's fight or flight.

Deep breathing also improves HRV (heart rate variability), the measurement of variance within intervals of the heart's beating (Bergland, 2017).

For ages, Eastern culture sages and yogis have understood and known about the importance of deep breathing. Western medicine practitioners today have accepted the importance of deep breathing as a core component of retaining and maintaining healthy physiological balance within the autonomic nervous system.

Breathing Technique, Method and Routine

Any kind of deep, slow breathing incorporating the diaphragm is going to stimulate your Vagus nerve, improve your HRV and activate the parasympathetic nervous system.

For some people, diaphragmatic breathing is a part of an everyday practice that is accompanied by customary mindfulness meditation or yoga. Other people simply deep breath anytime they feel stressed, angry or anxious in order to maintain control of their emotions and want to be relieved of these momentary emotions.

We take 10 to 14 breaths per minute on average. To stimulate the Vagus nerve, try breathing only 6 breaths per minute. Breathe in deeply and then breathe out slowly.

Some deep breathing methods recommend inhaling and exhaling only through the mouth. Other experts prescribe breathing only through the nose. Using a combination of both can also be applied. Whatever manner you feel comfortable with, feels right, and fits into your lifestyle is what's best for you individually.

All of these methods of diaphragmatic breathing can be incredibly beneficial.

In order for deep breathing to be consistently beneficial to stimulate the Vagus nerve, it should be practiced daily, at least once a day. Whatever breathing technique is right for you can be done in as little as 60 seconds anytime and anywhere.

Three cycles of inhaling and exhaling (three breaths in and three breaths out) can be extremely beneficial and you can do more if you are so inclined (Bergland, 2017).

Cold Exposure Therapy

Cold showers or rinse-offs, as well as dunking your face in cold water can stimulate the Vagus nerve. Studies have shown that your parasympathetic system (rest and relax) increases, facilitated by the Vagus nerve while your sympathetic system (fight or flight) decreases. According to a study, cold therapy also activates nitrergic neurons and cholinergic neurons through the nerve avenues.

All types of cold exposure, even having a drink of cold water helps to elevate the stimulating of the Vagus nerve. (Ropp, 2017)

Singing, Humming, and Chanting

Singing upbeat songs, singing hymns, mantra chanting, and humming all elevate your HRV in different ways. Singing initiates what you can call a "vagal pump" that sends out calming waves.

When you sing loudly, you're working the throat and back muscles activate the nerve. Singing with others, usually during church and synagogue services, also elevates Vagus function and HRV.

There is an increase in oxytocin when singing because people feel closer together when they sing.

Humming to a tune or OM during meditation also activates the Vagus as it sends out soothing waves to the nerve.

Prayer

Many religions have different ways of praying. Some chant, sing meditate, pray a Rosary to the rhythmic prayer of Judaism. It's good for your health and the vibrations in the throat stimulate the Vagus nerve.

Gargling

Who knew that something we do to protect our throat from bacteria and infection when we gargle could also be a remedy for low vagal tone? The muscles of the pallet are stimulated, which in turn activates the Vagus nerve.

When gargling, some patients will have tears well up in their eyes. This is a good sign. If this doesn't happen, it's recommended that the gargling be done regularly each day until they are able to tear up a bit. This immediately improves working memory function.

Laughing

Who doesn't like to laugh? Being able to laugh and having happiness in your life naturally boosts your immune system. Laughing also stimulates the Vagus nerve and increases HRV.

Sometimes people faint from laughing. This may be caused by the nerve becoming overstimulated (Ropp, 2017).

Massage

Massaging the neck can stimulate the Vagus nerve.

Having your feet massaged helps lower your blood pressure and heart rate. A pressure massage also activates the Vagus nerve as well as relaxes the body and works the muscles and the tissues.

Stomach Massage

Research shows that a massage of the stomach can lessen inflammation and tranquilizes the sensory system. A self-stomach massage has appeared to activate the Vagus nerve, progress insulin release to help equalize glucose in babies who are pre-term.

The combination of manual physical control and stimulation of the nerve can offer surprising benefits.

VAGUS NERVE

A frequent massage can give you an overall sense of relaxation, stimulates the Vagus nerve, and gives you a restful sleep.

Exercise

Your brain's growth hormone is increased when you exercise, supports the mitochondria of the brain and helps in the reversal of cognitive decline. It also stimulates the Vagus nerve and is beneficial for the brain and mental health. Gut flow is stimulated by mild exercise which is facilitated by the Vagus nerve.

When we move, the digestive system the peristaltic wave moves stool through the colon is activated and the digestive system is stimulated.

The movement is partially controlled by the Vagus nerve, which is also stimulated by exercise, from yoga, CrossFit or walking.

Exercise with whatever works for you is good to get started. Try to incorporate at least 15-30 minutes daily.

Tai Chi and Qi Gong

Stress activates the sympathetic system. The state of the body is in fight or flee reaction and the body faces stress and attack or runs away. Adrenalin is released into the body, heightened blood pressure and increased heart rate.

Relaxation is theVagus nerve being stimulated. This is when there is a regeneration of tissue and the body is at rest. Breathing is concentrated and the intention is to relax. Both aid in activating the nerve.

Major parts of Tai Chi and Qi Gong practice are slow, concentrated breathing, and the purpose is to relax. It is known that these two practices stimulate the Vagus nerve.

Adding the stretching and light spiraling movements to the breathing for the purpose of relaxing activates the alkaline response. This further aid the regeneration of tissue and internal healing. (Earth Balance Tai Chi, 2018)

Yoga, Mindfulness, Meditation, and Pranayama

Researchers who have been studying the impactful mind-body effects of yoga, mindfulness, meditation, and pranayama (breathing practices) have discovered it to be a key factor in activating the Vagus nerve.

This is the nerve of emotion impacting whether you feel safe and protected in a grounded, secure place. This is why practices that affect the nerve can feel their state of mind, and their sense of comfort improve while diminishing inflammation and stress.

We recognize that low vagal tone is an indication of stress and is typified by negativity, anxiety, depression, weak digestion, and inflammation. One's ability to manage stress, have psychological well-being and a balanced disposition is how optimal vagal tone is exemplified.

It is essential to elevate the vagal tone.

Yoga, mindfulness meditation and breathing have a powerful impact on vagal tone. A study with 35 test subjects practiced mindfulness meditation to manage stress, specifically unemployment, a truly stressful situation to be in.

The test was conducted for four months. After the four months, the subjects exhibited lowered inflammation and higher levels of brain connectivity, indicating a healthy vagal tone. (Susan, 2018)

Meditation incorporates deep breathing which stimulates the Vagus nerve. Choose whatever meditation works for you. Some people like guided meditations, some like to focus on breathing. Make a daily habit of doing at least 2 minutes of meditation each day.

Yoga Poses

The combination of physical, spiritual and mental exercises that uses exercises, breathing methods and meditation is the definition of yoga. The main goal of yoga exercises is to create harmony in the body, mind, and environment.

An ancient art with origins in Asia, yoga has become popular around the world due to its benefits to mental and physical health.

Yoga provides the benefits of managing stress and anxiety, the promotion of cardiovascular health, increase of self-control and self-awareness, mental clarity, improved body balance and flexibility, weight loss, muscle relaxation.

Unlike some other forms of exercise, yoga gives a person the ability to practice it regardless of age or physicality. There is no requirement for high-intensity exercise.

Yoga poses can be adjusted to suit even people with physical limitations and the elderly. The most significant thing is to make sure you seek out a credible instructor and if you have any physical limitations or conditions that you communicate that so poses can be customized for your body.

Yoga Tips

An important interconnection between Western medicine and Kundalini yoga lies in their individual understanding of the significance of the health of the Vagus nerve in health and well-being.

The Vagus nerve has been referred to as the central tuning string of the body by ancient yogis because when its frequency vibrates at the proper frequency, the heart creates an electromagnetic field that is comprehensible and harmonious.

Kundalini yoga combines meditation, breathing exercise and physical movement that can stimulate the Vagus nerve.

Vagus nerve stimulation through non-invasive techniques such as yoga and including yoga postures, breathing exercises, and mindfulness meditations are exceptional for stimulating the Vagus nerve.

Kundalini yoga has been found beneficial in increasing physical consciousness.

Seek out a yoga teacher who instructs Kundalini yoga. For your own benefit, practicing early in the morning and no less than 40 days will be the most advantageous to get the most from the sessions.

A Kundalini yoga class usually begins with an introduction from the teacher. The actual workout will last 45 minutes, leading into

VAGUS NERVE

a 15-minute session of relaxing followed by 20-minute meditation, including mantra chanting.

When you're increasing your vagal tone, yoga's role is to increase your autonomic nervous system as well as your flexibility. Yoga teaches you how to adjust from your sympathetic and parasympathetic systems. Practicing yoga will help to stimulate your Vagus nerve.

The support of your mental and physical health is why yoga is thought to be a good practice to maintain.

Other yoga tips – Use a non-slip mat to avert slipping or becoming injured. Do not eat before practicing yoga or have a full stomach and stretch the muscles before beginning a session. Take off all jewelry, contact lenses and tie your hair up to avoid having it get in the way. Focus on your poses, breathing exercises and meditation in a quiet environment.

Acupuncture

Acupuncture, the ancient Chinese medicine treatment, may be beneficial in stimulating the Vagus nerve. The Vagus nerve has been stimulated with acupuncture for years and there are many commonly used points that stimulate improved Vagus function.

Studies show that ear or auricular acupuncture is especially stimulating for the Vagus nerve and can benefit:

- Cardiovascular regulation

- Respiratory regulation

- Gastrointestinal tract regulation

Eating Fish

Eating fish increases vagal activity and tone. We get into a calming parasympathetic mode more frequently eating small fish that have less heavy metals in them.

Fasting

Intermittent fasting and the reduction of calories both increase HRV in animals which indicates this to be a marker of vagal tone.

Although there are no clinical studies, some people claim that intermittent fasting enhanced their HRV.

One theory indicates the Vagus nerve might facilitate a reduction in metabolism when a person is fasting. The nerve senses a decline in blood glucose and a diminishing of chemical and mechanical stimuli from the gut. Vagus nerve impulses from the liver to the brain increases, slowing the metabolic rate according to the tested animal data. (Albina, NP, MPH, Victoria, 2019)

Chewing Gum

The gut hormone CCK appears to directly trigger vagal impulses in the brain. The ability of CCK to reduce food intake and appetite depends on the impulses from the Vagus nerve to and from the brain.

Chewing may help to increase CCK release. Chewing sugar-free is advised as most gum contains additives and artificial sweeteners that are not healthy.

Develop an Exercise Routine

VAGUS NERVE

There are many exercises to choose from to stimulate the Vagus nerve. Whether you simply want to do breathing exercises or be more physical and adventurous and try yoga or Tai Chi, the most important exercise you can do is any one of them.

Many of us had never heard of the Vagus nerve and how impactful and vital it is to our body. Now that you know how vital it is to our body's functions, it makes sense to decide which exercises would make sense for you.

If you identify with many of the illnesses and diseases that stimulating the Vagus nerve can improve then it's time to act.

Create a routine all your own, work it around your daily schedule, and stick with it. A daily exercise routine will soon become second nature and you'll begin to feel and see the changes it makes.

Remember, the breathing exercises can be done anytime and anywhere and don't take more than 60 seconds. Nothing can be more convenient and less time consuming than this exercise.

Whatever you do, pay attention to your body, treat it with care, and get your Vagus nerve functioning at its optimum level for better health.

CONCLUSION

Thank you for making it through to the end of Vagus Nerve, let's hope it was informative and able to provide you with all of the tools you need to achieve your goals whatever they may be.

In an ideal world, we would be free of ailments and disease, but in reality, our bodies are subject to external and internal threats that ultimately influence on our physical health and mental wellbeing. This is what necessitates the autonomic nervous system to trigger responses that are appropriate to the prevailing conditions. Both the internal body environment and external surroundings.

Our greatest weapons against ill health and physical disorders ultimately lie in our understanding of how our body functions and in what way we can improve natural mechanisms to make it even more effective in self-renewal and repair. It is for this reason that we have gone through the Vagus nerve and its functions in the body as relates to good health.

By fully comprehending the healing potential that is contained in the vagus nerve, you have equipped yourself with the knowledge that will guide in taking a more natural approach to maintaining a healthy body. When we work together with our natural instincts and reflexes, we reap more in terms of creating the right homeostatic balance for body organs and processes to function.

Your understanding of the importance of vagal activity puts you in a unique position to change your outcomes and start living a healthier and happier life. We may not be able to avoid all illnesses and infections, but we can certainly reduce the frequency and severity of the disorders we routinely have to face.

The vagus nerve plays a crucial role in your overall health, and by taking the initiative to learn how it functions and how you can activate it, you have started your journey to unleashing your body's natural self-healing powers.

The next step is to start applying the techniques that you have learned in this book and following the guidelines provided consistently to achieve the best vagal tone possible, which will, in turn, translate into numerous health benefits for you.

Dr. Jason Rosenberg

Printed in Great Britain
by Amazon